Sky Don't Rain Daddy

Lionel Wilkes

First published in Great Britain by
Pen Press Publishers Ltd
39-41 North Road
Islington
London N7 9DP

ISBN 1 900796 98 8

A catalogue record of this book is available from
the British Library

Cover design by
Bridget Tyldsley

Sky Don't Rain Daddy

Lionel Wilkes

Pen Press Publishers Ltd
London

Dedication

I dedicate this book to our son Ian with love and affection.
To my wife Margaret who took on the most of the problems
of looking after Ian, and without whose help this book could not
have been written.
To Roy and Julie for being such great kids and giving us four
wonderful grandchildren. I love them all.

CHAPTER ONE

The one thing no parent should have to do is outlive their child. When your child dies, it is not possible to describe your feelings of guilt and anguish. In your mind, you constantly relive your life together. The worst times for me are the small hours of the morning, when I lie there awake, thinking: Could we have done more to revive him on that last morning? Then other thoughts come crowding in. Should we have spent more time with him? Helped and amused him more? Margaret was always so patient with Ian, while I would sometimes get angry and shout at him. That still haunts me seven years on.

Our son Ian was 35 years of age when he died. He was autistic, and had brain damage and severe epilepsy. This is Ian's story, with some of his family background thrown in. It's not all doom and gloom, far from it: among all the hassle there were plenty of happy times, things we still laugh about today.

Margaret and I got married on 25 July 1953 at Kings Norton Church and lived in one room at Hawksley Crescent in Northfield, Birmingham. When we had lived there for about 12 months, houses came off the ration and anyone could apply to buy one. So we put our name down and paid a deposit of £95 on a new Mucklows house in Hasbury, Halesowen. The total price was £1495. We moved into Bassanage Road in the Spring of 1955.

Early in 1956 Margaret told me we were expecting a baby. When the time came, Margaret was late going into labour so, on the doctor's advice, she went into the Mary Steven's Nursing Home

1

for the baby to be induced. They did this with injections in those days. If this did not start the birth, she would have had to go into the maternity hospital at Loveday Street in Birmingham. Margaret had the injections, but Ian was born too fast. This meant that the doctors had trouble getting him to breathe, and he had to go into an oxygen tent for some hours till he stabilised. This was in the early hours of 15 December 1956, exactly one week after Margaret's birthday.

The weather had turned nasty early that year. As we only had a motorcycle in those days, it was a struggle for me to go and see mother and baby through the snow and ice every night. They kept Margaret and Ian in for eight days and I got a taxi to bring them home. As we said goodbye to the nurses, one of them said, 'We never thought we would save you, my love' as she kissed Ian. Little did we know how traumatic his life and ours were to be. Ian was a lovely looking baby and a real cherub as he lay gurgling away in his cot those first few months.

Ian was Christened in Halesowen. We had the top tier of our wedding cake for the party and a lot of home-made beer. (In those days every corner shop in the Black Country sold hops and malt for home brewers and a lot of homes still had a brew house in the garden.)

Everything seemed to be going well. Ian was a good baby and we were so proud, but the clouds were on the horizon. Margaret had a friend Brenda who lived in Halesowen. She had a baby girl the same age as Ian, but she seemed brighter and more alert than Ian. When Margaret asked the doctor about it he said, 'Don't compare him with other children, they're all different'. Looking back, Margaret always had a feeling that all was not well. Time was to prove her right.

It was this sort of comment that we heard repeatedly over the coming years, as the medical profession didn't believe Margaret or me. They seemed to be of the opinion that all parents are too fussy to be objective and always exaggerate. It happened again when Ian started to have convulsions. They told us this time that it was only because he was teething, the same 'we know best' attitude that we were subjected to all through Ian's life.

Soon our boy's behaviour changed. He yelled and screamed a lot. Also, his violent side-to-side rocking started. He seemed to be in a lot of pain, but it baffled our doctor. Ian became increasingly difficult to cope with. At that time there was an old man who used to sit outside his son's shop in Hasury. He would give the local children a sweet when they went past after school. When Margaret used to go past with Ian in the pram, he was often screaming. So the old fellow told Margaret to get a good piece of gristle from the butcher, tie it on a piece of string and let Ian chew it. 'It always worked with my young uns,' he said. We didn't try it but we did get Ian a dummy; he got through two or three a day. So perhaps a piece of gristle would have lasted longer!

About this time we moved house and bought a country grocery store. We were hoping to build a new life for ourselves. Looking back, it was a crazy thing to do, but we were young and immature and, as they say, you can't put an old head on young shoulders. The property consisted of two cottages, each with two rooms up and two down, and a toilet halfway down the garden. The one cottage we let at a controlled rent of six shillings and four pence a week (about 33p in new money). The front room of our cottage had the shop in it and this opened directly onto the main road. There were four more cottages in the block.

The village, Dayhouse Bank, consisted of thirty three cottages, our shop, a pub and the chapel. To the side of the cottages we had a plot of land, about half an acre with deep litter chicken houses on it. This had planning permission for a new shop and dwelling. We had to learn how to run a shop and, as I was working six days a week, most of it fell on Margaret's shoulders. With Ian being so difficult, we were beginning to find life very hard, so we decided to employ someone to help Margaret during the day. This was how Mrs Lucy Maguire came into our life. She still corresponds with us over forty years later. She had eight children and helped with Ian as well as in the shop.

The walls between the cottages were so thin that you could hear everything that went on next door. You even knew when someone broke wind. Ian was at his most difficult during this period, so it was amazing that we never had a word of complaint from either side. At this time he screamed all day and all night and the only way we could calm him was to have him on our laps in a rocking chair. So I used to rock him till about 2am while Margaret got some sleep. Then she would take over while I got my sleep. I had to be at work at 7.30am, so neither of us got much rest during this time in Ian's life.

Looking back, I wonder how we did manage. Margaret was a mother in a million but if she had not had Lucy to help her, I am sure she would have cracked up. To make matters worse, I had started to build an extension to the rear of the cottage, to provide a kitchen, flush toilet and septic tank. I dug all the footings and the septic tank by hand, and employed a man named Martindale to do the brickwork and plastering. I did the plumbing and electrical work myself. I was, after all, an electrician at the Austin Motor Company. It all seemed worthwhile when we were able to go to the toilet without having to go halfway down the garden to the earth closet with a double seat. This made us the proud owners of the second flush toilet in Dayhouse Bank. We also had the advantage of a new kitchen with hot water on tap.

Flushed with my DIY success, I got the draughtsman in the electronics lab where I worked to do some drawings for the new shop and house. When we got the drawings passed I started work once again, digging footings, drainage and septic tank by hand. Only this time I had a gang of bricklayers working weekends for cash in hand. It was not long after I'd started the new house that Margaret told me I was about to become a father again. So we must have spent some quality time together although, looking back, I can't figure out how we found the time or energy!

Living in Dayhouse Bank was like going back 100 years in time. The local people never grumbled about Ian. On the one hand, they were very tolerant and would give you anything, although they didn't have much to give. At the same time, some of them would pinch the sugar out of your tea. Ian would throw toys and garden things over the hedge at the bottom of the garden. When I saw him do it, I would run through the shop, down the road and round the back lane. But whenever I got there, whatever he had thrown over would have disappeared, and nobody in sight.

There were plenty of characters for such a small place. There was an old chap called Lank Wood who said that children could always learn to swear, no matter how young. As Ian was not talking yet, Lank would try and get him to swear. Ian was four years old before he began to talk and his first words were 'sod it', so it seemed that Lank was right!

One woman used to come into the shop every lunchtime and have a large bottle of pop, a tin of salmon or corned beef and a block of ice-cream or chocolate. With the lack of washing facilities, she had not had a bath for years, so every time she came into the shop we had to open the door and window to let in some fresh air. This particular customer came in every day for her usual lunch. At about 5 pm she would come back and ask for a tin of Goblin Stew for 'the Bleeder's' tea, as she often called her husband. This went on for about six weeks, then one night she came back into the shop with Goblin Stew running all down her. She said, 'Give us summat else for his tea, the bleeder's tired of stew.'

This same lady purchased a new coat from the tally man before Christmas, to wear to her niece's wedding at Easter. She wore it every day, even carried the coal for the fire in it. She came into the shop the day before the wedding and asked for a packet of Omo, stoked the copper up, and boiled her coat in it. She went to the wedding the next day with the coat still dripping! So you can see we always had something to laugh about.

At least everyone helped in an emergency, like the Sunday a couple of years later, that Ian disappeared. He was about four years old at the time. One minute he was there, then he had gone. The trouble was that Ian did not respond when you called him or spoke to him. So it was no use calling him, you just had to find him. Within ten minutes of our missing him, the whole village was out looking, all the adults and the children. So with all this help we found him in about half an hour. He was running down the hedgerow in a nearby field after crossing a busy road. Mind you, it felt like half a day, not half an hour.

By the time that Roy was born on 9 January 1959, Ian had become quieter but was still very difficult. He used to rock from side to side, screaming if you tried to hold or cuddle him. He was also hyperactive, which made him very difficult to cope with. Roy was such a pleasure to us after all Ian's problems. It was nice to be able to really enjoy having him. With a child like Ian, you gradually find that your friends stop coming to see you, and make excuses if you suggest calling to see them. So another problem arose as our whole family became isolated. Often furniture and plants would be thrown across the room or tipped over whenever you took your eyes off Ian. I had to screw everything down to prevent this. He would bite and kick when he came near anyone; it was a wonder that little Roy survived. The district nurse said to Roy, after our daughter Julie was born, 'I'll never know how we reared you, my love.'

The lack of help and support for families like us in the late 50s and through the 60s was total. Although we were seeing the doctor and going to the children's hospital, no one came to see how we were coping or gave us advice on how to cope. Yet somehow we managed.

With the building work on the new house now at the brickwork stage, Ian was able to vent his frustrations on the odd bricks and piles of sand lying around on the building site. That summer he started to sleep better, so I went on to the night shift. I could get more work done on the new building, and at least I could have Ian with me in the afternoons to help Margaret out.

We now had an A35 van that I had purchased through the employees' scheme at work. We got a good discount. We fitted seats in the back so it now had four. Later that summer, I drove past the new building in the early morning on my way home from work. I sensed something was wrong, so I went back and saw that lightning had struck the scaffolding during the night. It had brought down the whole gable end of the building, so we had to order more bricks and start to rebuild. Unfortunately we had not insured the new building, so it was a hard way to learn our lesson. This caused a cash-flow problem that delayed our progress, as we had to save like mad to make up the deficit. The snow and ice during the following winter held things up even further, but by next spring we were back in full swing.

Roy was by now out of his pram and into everything, enjoying messing about on the site with Ian. One day I jumped off the scaffold onto a plank of wood with a nail stuck through it, and when I picked my foot up the plank came with it. They say things happen in threes: well, they did this time, as Margaret trod on a nail the next week, then, blow me, Roy did the same a couple of days later! So we had a great purge and cleared the site.

We had decided that running the shop and looking after Ian and Roy was getting too difficult, so we asked the council if we could sell the shop and move into the new house. They said no, they had given planning permission for a new shop, not a private residence. This meant we would have to sell the new building, which we did in 1962. We sold it to my parents, who had been running a cafe in Cofton Park near Rednal, in the Lickey Hills. The lease had just run out and they had to find somewhere else. So Mom now ran the country stores village shop from the new property and we had more time to concentrate on Ian and Roy.

In 1961 we exchanged our van for a Nash Metropolitan car. The Austin Motor Company made them for Nash in America. As a consequence, not many were sold in the UK. They were lovely little cars, with a bench seat across the front and two small seats in the back, very American looking. They were always in two colours, black & white, green & white, and so on. Ours was red & white. We then decided to go on holiday, and booked a caravan in a field miles from anywhere, so Ian would not disturb anyone. We all had a lovely time, especially Roy, with trips to Weston-Super-Mare and Cheddar.

We had been back at home for a few months when an old lady who was a neighbour, a Mrs Lambert, died. She had lived in a little old bungalow to the rear of a shop (now named The Chalet). We still have a carver chair we bought from her for 10 shillings (50p). A little while after she died we purchased the bungalow for £1000 from her son. Before moving in we constructed an extension to provide a better kitchen and bathroom. We used the old kitchen as a dining room. I had to make the table with bench seats and screw them to the floor and wall to stop Ian throwing them through the window. We moved in and sold our cottage to my sister Margot and her husband Tony.

CHAPTER TWO

At the bungalow we had three-quarters of an acre of garden. As it was on a steep bank, I terraced it so I could have a vegetable patch. I also built a playhouse up in the air on poles and made a strong swing for Ian and Roy to play with. Every day I came home wondering what repairs I would have to do that night. Usually it would only be reglazing a window or replanting part of the garden. However, sometimes I would have to fit a new toilet or cistern. Ian had a habit of hiding things inside the cistern or jamming them down the toilet pan, usually his own toys but on one occasion he put Roy's goldfish down the loo.

He also had no sense of danger and would walk along the window sills, or on the outhouse roof. He would climb up there to stuff things down the chimney to the old copper. One minute he would be with you, the next you would look out of the dining room window and see Ian on the outhouse roof, so it was panic stations once again. We had a lot of rats in the garden at the time and as Ian was into everything, I could not put poison down or set breakback traps. I could only set cage traps to catch them. It was quite disconcerting to see a group of four or five rats looking down into the dining room watching you eat your food, so they had to go.

On one occasion we had to take Ian to the children's hospital in Birmingham as he had ruptured himself throwing the furniture about. That was an extremely hair-raising experience. Although Ian could still not talk, he could let you know he was not very happy. He would throw himself and anything he could get his hands on about,

9

while screaming the place down. The average waiting time was about two hours, and all the other people waiting would be saying things like 'He wants a good hiding' and 'You should be ashamed, letting him carry on like that.' The doctor told us that Ian needed an operation and that the waiting time would be about two years. We had to go to and from the hospital by bus, as the car was in for repair after I'd had a bump in it. On the way home Margaret cried. She was very upset, saying Ian would not survive for two years.

This made us consider our options and we decided the only thing to do was to see a specialist privately. We managed to get an appointment very quickly and made the journey to his surgery in Edgbaston. There was no waiting this time and after the doctor had examined Ian, he said our son would require the operation as soon as possible. He then asked me what I did for a living and how much I earned. I told him, and he said he would do the operation on the national health within the next two weeks. I worried about Ian ripping the scar open again, so I asked the doctor about it. He said that Ian might rupture himself somewhere else but not in the same place.

Ian was in hospital ten days later for his operation. In those days, parents could not see their children while they were in hospital; the medical staff thought it would upset the children too much. When we went to get Ian after his operation, the nurse told us that he had bitten a nurse. He had taken a lump out of her arm and she had ended up in hospital herself. We said how sorry we were, but they told us not to worry, it was all part of the job. What a job!

The shock of being in hospital started Ian talking. When he came out and we took him up to the shop to see his nanny, he tripped over the doorstep and said his first words: 'Oh, sod it!' It amused and amazed us, as this was the first time he had spoken. From then on he began to use more words but never talked very well.

Ian was not screaming all the time now, but he still had screaming sessions, and his other problems made life more difficult for the rest of the family. Some things made us laugh, however, like when he found a pair of scissors we had not hidden away. Ian went quiet for a short time, which made us wonder what he was up to. When we found him, he had cut all the hair off one side of his head, as well as his eyelashes and eyebrows on the one side. Margaret now had to try and make him look presentable by cutting off the rest of his hair. It seemed such a shame, as he was a lovely looking boy. Still, at least hair grows fast when you are five years old.

At work we had very relaxed working conditions, as we were working on developing new control gear for machine tools. We were always teasing the apprentices. One of the things we did was to put up a small prize of half a crown (12½ p) for whoever could hold an electric soldering iron the longest time after we switched it on. We would roll about laughing, watching their expressions as the irons got hotter. Some of the things we had done to us, and things we got up to when we were apprentices would not bear repeating, even in this enlightened age.

I was able to get some light relief at work, but Margaret was in the deep end all the time. I still wonder to this day how she coped. The winter was the worst, as we seemed to have more snow for longer periods than the rest of the country. This meant she was stuck in the house with all the problems of occupying Ian and Roy.

As 1962 approached, Roy was three years old. Being constantly in Ian's company, he was starting to copy his older brother's behaviour. We decided that we would have to do something about it and looked into sending both Ian and Roy to school. This meant we would have to consider a private school. We got them into Greenmore College in Edgbaston for the summer term. They both looked so sweet in their school uniforms as they set off for their first day. Roy settled in straight away but the staff had problems with Ian. They could not get him into the school. They had to put a table and chair outside and keep him there all day. Luckily the weather was fine all that week!

However, this state of affairs could not continue so we had to stop taking Ian. This meant that Margaret had to take Roy into Birmingham to school every day and have Ian at home. It was all worthwhile as Roy thrived at school, and he stopped copying Ian. During the summer we looked into other schools for Roy and finally settled on Whitford Hall in Bromsgrove. It was the best thing we ever did, as the headmistress and staff liked Roy, and thought the sun shone out of his backside.

Around this time the Department of Education contacted us about Ian's education. They made an appointment to see us and sent someone to assess Ian. After trying to get him to do a lot of puzzles, they told us to send him to hospital and forget him as he would never improve. You can imagine the devastating effect this had on us, but we told them what they could do with their advice, and soldiered on.

It was also about this time that we joined the local Mencap Society, who informed us about the day centre in Bromsgrove. We made inquiries and Ian started to go daily. For a little while all seemed well, as at last Margaret was getting a break during the day. This was just the lull before the storm, however, for out of the blue they told us that they would not allow Ian to continue at the day centre. We wanted to know why. They told us that when Ian misbehaved, and they locked him in the cloakroom, he pulled all the coats off the pegs. This comment made us angry.

So Ian was back home all the time again. There was no respite care in those days, or if there was they kept it very quiet. Although Ian was still very difficult this was probably his brightest time. He knew some of his colours and could count a little. But he was developing other bad habits. He started to chew the arms of his jumpers, and if you left him for a few minutes, he would rip the arm off completely. He had started to bite himself when he got upset. Being at home all the time was having a negative effect on him. He was getting more and more withdrawn as the winter dragged on.

Finally we got Ian an appointment to have a scan at the hospital in Birmingham. The day that we took him there was a nightmare. He had to keep still during the scan. He screamed and fought the staff, making them take a long time to get a result. Ian was upset when we got home and he vented his anger on the door, smashing it off its hinges. It's no wonder our friends and relatives used to look on in amazement at his antics. Margaret let it all pass over her head; if she hadn't, I think she would have ended up in hospital herself! As she said, he could be magic to be with at times, and even when he was having one of his tantrums, we would often have a good laugh when things quietened down.

Early in 1963 we were getting more and more worried about Ian, and kept trying to get some advice. We finally got an appointment to see a Dr Patterson at Lea Hospital in Bromsgrove. This was a special hospital for the mentally handicapped. We tried to get Ian into the hospital to see the doctor but he played up so much that we had to take him back to the car. I went in to see Dr Patterson and told him what had happened. He was fantastic and said he would come out to the car to see Ian. When he sat by Ian and started to try and talk with him, Ian promptly bit him, but the doctor was not the least bit upset. He arranged for Ian to attend the special school at Lea Castle Hospital in Kidderminster on a daily basis. This meant Margaret taking Roy to school at Bromsgrove, then driving Ian to Lea Castle, a round trip of 45 miles. Then in the afternoon she had to collect Ian, then go back to Bromsgrove to collect Roy, a further 45 miles. This went on five days a week for years. It's no wonder that, with all that experience, Margaret is a better driver than me!

The year rolled by. Roy was enjoying school and was a favourite pupil at Whitford Hall. Ian was still biting and ripping his clothes. In July he had a fall and broke his arm. When we took him to Bromsgrove hospital he got very upset while we were waiting to see the doctor. He was squealing non stop, upsetting the rest of the people waiting. The staff were excellent, so very understanding. This was such a rare occurrence that it made Margaret happy but also sad when she thought of most people's attitude. When we took Ian back to have his plaster off, the sister did it in the car as Ian got so upset again. This was the sort of thing that made life bearable. Kind people can really be a blessing and comfort in this cruel world.

About this time Margaret had some good news for us: we were going to have another baby in March. As summer turned to Autumn, there was also some bad news. Roy's class teacher said that she thought he was deaf, as he did not seem to hear much of what she said. We took him to the doctor, who sent us to see a specialist at Bromsgrove Hospital. He said that Roy had a rigid ear drum, caused by pressure inside the ear. It would mean making a hole in the ear drum to let the pressure out. At the same time he would remove Roy's tonsils and adenoids.

When we saw Roy after the operation, he looked such a poor mite, we wondered if we had done the right thing. The only food he could swallow was ice cream. He was very poorly for several days, but then he came on in leaps and bounds. When he went back at school, he soon became top of his class.

Ian, however, was not improving at all. He still knew some colours and could count up to ten most of the time, but his behaviour was still very difficult. That winter Margaret knitted some balaclavas for Ian. As soon as you took your eyes off him he would stuff them down the toilet and flush them away or throw them on the fire. We lost count of the hats Margaret knitted that winter.

Ian had a lot of obsessions. When he fell down the septic tank, he kept insisting Margaret did drawings of it. Woe betide Margaret if some small detail was not identical to those in the previous drawings! After a few weeks it would be something else that preoccupied him. He also loved music, some tunes more than others. He loved most of the Beatles' music, though there was one tune he hated, 'A Hard Day's Night'.

Ian's seventh birthday came around, then Roy's fifth. Margaret was looking very pregnant now, and early in march she went to Bromsgrove Hospital to have the baby. True to our form, things did not go smoothly. I think the sister was the model for the Carry On films: a real battle-axe. I tried to explain to her how Ian's problems had arisen but she he had no interest in what we were saying. She said, 'We know what we are doing.' We had learnt over the years that this was the time to worry. Again we were right, as things got worse. Margaret caught the flu and when Julie was born, the staff put them both in a side ward. Any woman who has given birth will have some idea of what Margaret went through, giving birth while suffering from flu.

Back home I was looking after Ian and Roy. The morning that Margaret had Julie I woke up at about 5am, feeling awful. I also had the flu and as I lay there I thought: if I die now I will at least be at peace. By 6am I managed to wake Roy and get him to come in to me. I was so weak that I could not get out of bed.

Roy was a real trooper. He was only just five years old but he got dressed himself. During the night we'd had a foot of snow, so he had to struggle up the hill through the snow to get his nanny out of bed. I will never know how the little mite managed. The doctor could not get through to see me, so Dad had to walk to Rubery to get some medicine for me. So there we were: Margaret in hospital with the flu and a new baby, and me stuck at home in bed with the flu, unable to visit them. But when I finally got to Bromsgrove and saw Julie for the first time, I realised it had all been worthwhile.

Not long after Margaret came home with Julie, we took Ian to see Dr Patterson at Lea hospital for one of his rare check-ups. This was when they told us for the first time that Ian was autistic. At this time very few people had heard of autism, including many doctors.

CHAPTER THREE

Once we were aware of the existence of autism, it became quite clear that Ian had all the typical symptoms. If you tried to hug or cuddle him, he would go as stiff as a board. If you did a drawing, it had to be the same as the one before, and the one before that. If we did not do everything to a strict routine, any deviation, however small, led to an outburst from Ian. So we tended to go along with his wishes: anything for an easy life. However, we still had plenty of upsets, and we did not have a clue what caused most of them. I was now doing another spell on nights, so I could help a bit with taking Roy and Ian to school.

I was going across the common to work one night when I saw a baby tawny owl in the road. As it was getting dark, I thought he would get run over so I put him in the car and took him home next morning. He soon became a permanent fixture, and we called him Tawny. Roy and I would mince up steak to feed him with. After adding the hair we had collected from combing the cat and dog, we also added our own nail clippings to make it more like the food he would get in the wild. I made a pen in the old outside toilet. When we had reared him to adulthood, we had to train him to hunt. We did this by tying a piece of meat to some string, and letting Tawny chase it. He soon learnt how to do it, and would go off to find his own food; but he always came back when I called him. We got a lot of pleasure out of Tawny. I soon learned to wear a leather jacket, as he would draw blood when he landed on my arm, even through my shirt.

Early the next year, Tawny started to call out and soon a female owl started to call back to him. Then he went off courting, but would always come back. Then the inevitable happened. He went off one night and never came back to me. Although he was nesting in the garden, I knew he was OK as he would answer me when I called him. I was glad that he went back to the wild, but we did miss him.

Well, back to the family. My mother was a Raybold and most of them had auburn hair. Julie kept up the family tradition, as her hair was like burnished copper. So she was a great favourite with her nanny. Our children missed out in some ways as Margaret's mother had died when Margaret was only twelve. She'd also lost her dad when she was seventeen. This meant that our children only had one set of grandparents. It also meant that Margaret did not have her mom to help her through the difficult times we had over the years with Ian. My mother was not able to help much as she was busy in the shop from early in the morning till seven in the evening. But she was a big help when Julie was a little older, and started to get carsick. Margaret was still travelling ninety miles a day on the school runs, which caused a problem, as Julie suffered from car sickness. So Mom started to look after Julie while Margaret was taking Ian and Roy to school.

This was a little in the future, so back to 1964. Early in the summer I took Roy camping. We pitched our tent at the bottom of Snowdon, and as I had not been camping before it was an adventure for both of us. We camped not far from the railway that ran up Snowdon. As the fare was expensive, I decided we would walk up to the top and ride back down. By the time we were halfway up, we were both exhausted. So after a long rest and our picnic lunch, we made our way back to camp. So much for our dreams of emulating Hillary and Tensing on Everest! But it was a nice holiday for both of us.

We were in for another shock. We received a letter informing us that the new M5 was going to be built up the valley behind our bungalow. The letter informed us that five yards across the bottom of our garden was going to be compulsorily purchased and - wait

17

for it - they offered us the princely sum of £10 compensation! When I complained they told me, 'You have nothing to complain about, we pay the legal charges.' Then, when the surveyors began work, I came home to find that the route they were pegging out was heading straight for our bungalow. They had chopped down the hedge and some trees, and after a lot of argument, they realised that the property to be demolished was the pair of cottages next door. We never did get an apology for the damage they had done.

They do say there is some good in everything. When construction of the road started, Mom did a roaring trade in the shop. It was the only shop within miles, and all the workers came in for their bacon butties and food for lunch. For months we had huge earth movers roaring up and down from six in the morning till eight at night. While the construction of the motorway was going on, my brother and I purchased a plot of land two doors up from the shop. We had some drawings done and passed by the council, and started to build a house to sell. We did the heavy work ourselves and subcontracted the brickwork and other skilled work.

Ian was still very overactive and taking up most of Margaret's attention. In late 1964, when Julie was crawling around and getting into everything, something happened. We were not sure what, but when I came home from work, Margaret said, 'I think Julie has had a fall, because every time I touch or try to pick her up she screams.' We had to take her to the doctor, so we put Ian and Roy into the car with us. Luckily Ian liked going in the car, and this took much of the stress out of travelling with him.

When we arrived the doctor saw us straight away. He examined Julie but did not know what the trouble was. He fetched his colleagues and they still had no idea what the trouble was, so he advised us to take her to the Children's Hospital in Birmingham. The trouble with having a child like Ian is that every time one other child has something wrong with them, it's panic stations all the way. So it seemed a long journey, although it was only about twelve miles.

At the hospital, they still could not decide what was wrong with Julie, so they sent for the consultant. When she arrived she was not very happy, as she had been in the middle of her dinner. She took one look at Julie and said, 'Have you taken this child's temperature?' No one had. When they took her temperature it was 103°. She had tonsillitis. So it was a course of antibiotics and Julie was back to normal.

Everything was still a hell of a rush every morning. Margaret had to get Julie ready to go to her nanny's, then Ian and Roy ready for school. It was lucky that Roy quickly learned to wash and dress himself, as this was a great help to Margaret.

This particular day was one of those mornings when everything seems to go wrong. Margaret had suddenly noticed that Ian was missing, and when she went outside to look for him she heard lots of horns tooting on the motorway. It had been open for a few months and was getting quite busy in the mornings. Margaret ran down the garden towards the motorway. She was horrified to see Ian walking up the middle of the northbound motorway, with the cars and trucks swerving around him and hooting their horns furiously. Not one tried to stop and see what the problem was. Margaret had to run up the side of the road, then run across and grab him. When she got back home, Roy had come up trumps again. He was looking after Julie like an older child, not a 5-year old.

After this incident we managed to get the Ministry of Transport to put a proper fence along our garden, instead of the posts with three strands of wire which they had initially insisted was safe enough. It would be lovely to have the experience and wisdom you get by the time you draw your pension. With the knowledge we have now, we could have made some of the civil servants and medical people stand up and take notice. I suppose it only comes from experience.

Up to a certain point in Ian's life, Ian always insisted that he was a 'cottage boy'. That was when we lived in the cottage; but when we moved to the bungalow it was 'Ian is a bungalow boy'. If you happened to mention anything about a cottage, Ian would get into a real state, shouting, 'Ian is not a cottage boy!' and jumping up and down. Even when he was not there we found ourselves being very careful and picking our words to avoid saying the wrong thing. Poor Ian, he must have felt so insecure.

Christmas 1964 came and, as usual, the family came to have dinner with us, mainly because Ian only felt secure and settled in his own home. You could not say content, as he very rarely was.

At this point I should mention that my father had a fear of spending money all his life. Consequently he had never bought anyone a present in his life. I remember when I was demobbed from the army, I didn't want to see my uniform again, so Dad wore it to work for years, even though he was three inches taller than me. This meant that the trousers were too short, or 'half mast', as Mom would say.

Any road up, as we say in the Midlands, to get back to that Christmas. When everyone came to dinner, Dad gave me a parcel, much to my surprise. I asked what it was, and he said, 'It's a present for Julie.' I nearly died on the spot. When I got my breath back I asked, 'Where are Ian's and Roy's?' He said he hadn't got them anything, so I told him he couldn't buy for one and not the others. After that, he always bought a Christmas present for all his grandchildren, as long as it did not cost much. It's the thought that counts, I suppose.

The New Year came along and we were back into our routine, Margaret still driving 90 miles a day, knitting balaclavas and jumpers, trying to keep up with Ian's appetite for biting them to bits. She spent all her time amusing the children when they were home, and only doing the housework when they were in bed. Sometimes, long after midnight, I would get angry and say 'Why the hell can't you do it in the day?' but it made no difference. She just carried on and I had to accept it in the end. Looking back over the years, I can see why our children turned out so well, kids to be proud of. It was the quality time Margaret spent with them, even though Ian was so difficult.

I was still working at the Austin Motor Company and labouring on the new house David and I were building up the road, as well as gardening and working on our bungalow. It was a seven-day week. So that spring I took Roy to London for a break for both of us.

We did the sights, fed the pigeons in Trafalgar Square, visited the museums and went to the pictures. All in all, 1965 was an uneventful year, if the traffic building up on the motorway and Ian's problems could be called 'uneventful'.

We were starting to think about extending the bungalow, as we only had two bedrooms. We really needed two more, one for Julie and one to give Roy his own space away from Ian, as he couldn't keep anything safe from his older brother, who was still quite destructive. If left on his own he would break anything that came to hand, so poor Roy's things got broken, but he always took it well. As he said many years later, he got his own back by burying Ian's cars in the garden - and I thought he had developed an interested in gardening! Not that it mattered, as every time we took Ian out we bought him a new matchbox car. At that time in his life he insisted that the doors opened, and since not many models did it caused problems in the shops. He would play up, but we soon learned to carry a spare.

Ian was eight now and when we took him out, we had to hold his hand, as we did for the rest of his life. He was a tall, good-looking boy who looked older than his years, so when he played up, as he inevitably did, we got some very funny looks and remarks, such as, 'What he wants is a good hiding' and 'Spoilt brat'. I got angry about this, but Margaret got upset as well as angry. I have come to realise that there is little you can do about other people's intolerance. You just have to learn to live with it. I am sure they do not realise how small things like that make life harder for people like us.

Soon we entered another phase in Ian's life. Margaret and I were in the dining room with Ian one day when he went into an epileptic fit. Having no previous knowledge of epilepsy, I thought the main thing to do was to prevent the person having a fit from biting their tongue. So what did I do? I put my thumb between Ian's teeth. The pain was unbelievable, and I could not do a thing about it till the fit was over. When we took Ian to the doctor's, he told me that if I had put my thumb between Ian's front teeth instead of his back teeth, he could have bitten it off. So I had ended up with a thumb like something in a Tom and Jerry cartoon for a few days, but at least I still had a thumb.

The doctor put Ian on Phenobarbitone to try to control his fits. It may have made them less frequent, but it did not stop them. For the rest of his life it was one long battle trying to control his fits. The one side effect of the Phenobarbitone that we did come to notice was that Ian gradually became quieter and less active. This increased over time, and he lost what little ability he did have to count and remember his colours. It did not, however, effect his autistic symptoms and all those problems carried on.

So in addition to Ian's behavioural problems, we now had to contend with the added problem of him having several fits a week. This is quite frightening when you have no experience of epilepsy. To make matters worse, no one ever bothered to tell us about placing him in the recovery position, which we only found out about a few years later, and now know is essential.

Still, everyday life goes on. It was now obvious that we couldn't wait any longer to extend the bungalow. With Ian having fits in the night as well as the day, he was disturbing Roy's sleep. So we had some plans drawn and submitted to the council. As we all know well, the mills of God and councils grind very fine and slow, so it was late in 1965 before we got the go-ahead. After doing the donkey work myself I employed a bricklayer to start building. As the bungalow was on a slope, there was a lot of brickwork below damp course. He started after Christmas, but before he got to the damp course, we had some hard frosts. This went on for six weeks. Each week he came and asked me for some money from his total labour price. Although he had not been able to do any work, I have always been an easy touch so I paid him. By the time he could start work again, he had drawn most of the money. So off to Germany he went to earn big money. We had paid out most of the money for labour, and the work was not done. The bricklayer's father got embarrassed about it all, so he said he would do the work in his spare time, at no cost. We were pleased with him when he did the work, although it did make the job drag out, and I did pay him a little to show our gratitude. Finally we were decorating and Roy had his own room at last. We had extended the lounge with a small bedroom to the side. Roy's new room was in the roof space with his own little staircase. It was just the room for a young boy, his own den in the sky.

CHAPTER FOUR

As Margaret was driving so many miles every day, we had to change the car and we purchased a new Austin Mini. We got it through the worker's scheme, which meant we had a 16% discount off the full price. If I remember correctly we paid just over £400 for it, and petrol was around 6 shillings (30p) a gallon.

Ian's fits were still causing problems. He was having the whole range of fits, from absences through *petit mal* to *grand mal*. The thing that amazes me now is the fact that no one gave us any instructions on what to do in an emergency. With Ian going to Lea Castle in Kidderminster every day, it meant that he was on the spot when he needed an ECG (electrocardiogram), which checks the brainwave patterns to see if the doctors can find what causes the epilepsy. Not that this ever helped: Ian was still on Phenobarbitone, a very addictive drug.

Although they called it a school at Lea Castle, they never tried to teach anything other than social skills and craft work. Not that Ian was capable of any social skills. I think the main objective was to occupy the residents. Ian was probably the only one who went daily. As an example of Ian's vocal ability, Mrs Sandow, his teacher, told us that one day a visitor had asked Ian what he was doing. Ian thoroughly confused her when he told her that Fitzroy's mother was dead. Fitzroy was a coloured boy. He had been in the hospital since he was a baby and never had any visitors. Ian had got it into his head that Fitzroy's mother had died. Whether he had just assumed this or had heard something, we will never know, as Ian was not able to tell us.

Much later, when Fitzroy was about sixteen, the doctors who had always believed that he was mentally handicapped discovered that he was totally deaf, and not mentally handicapped at all. He had to stay at Lea Castle, as the deaf school said it was too late to start teaching him. It's the stuff that can give you nightmares, when you think what must have gone through his mind over the years. Fitzroy died before his seventeenth birthday from sickle-cell anaemia. And you thought fate had dealt you a bad hand.

That year we decided to try going on holiday. We booked a caravan on a farm near Weston, thinking that if we were in a caravan on our own, Ian might settle. The caravan was all alone in an orchard away from the farm, which made it ideal. Roy and Julie were able to play in the field and we went to the beach in Weston most days. Ian enjoyed playing in the sand with Roy and Julie, we had lovely weather, and Roy and I had a bonus when the farmer invited us in to watch England beat Germany in the World Cup final. (We have been waiting for a repeat ever since.) One day as we were playing football in the field outside the caravan, an RAF fighter plane flew overhead. There was a huge explosion, and when we looked up we saw two parachutes open. We ran over to where they were coming down and were just in time to see them land. One pilot landed safely, but the other broke his leg on landing. At least none of them was seriously hurt. It was a lovely holiday but we never seemed to be able to repeat it. We did try in subsequent years but it never worked out.

Back home things soon got back into the regular routine. Ian was still developing strange habits, though he still liked music. Sometimes we would buy the latest pop record or toy, and Ian would take an instant dislike to it, then insist on Margaret burying it in the garden. She always had to do this the same way every time, as if performing some pagan ceremony. Woe betide the person brave enough to change the pattern! Our problems with Ian made us worry about not being able to take Roy and Julie out as much as other families do. Not that Ian was always playing up, but he got so distressed when he was away from the security of home. Poor Ian, he must have felt awful. One of the problems with autism is that you cannot hold or hug sufferers to comfort them. They just go as stiff as a board, and do not respond in any way. So it meant that either Margaret took Roy and Julie out, and I looked after Ian, or the other way round. But most of the time we just stayed at home.

I was getting restless at work, thinking more about our building job and less about electronics, though we did have some fun, like the time we had a new driver to take us around the factory to maintain our equipment. His probation officer had found the job for him. The first morning he arrived for work, he came in a large car and parked just outside the lab. In the car were a dollybird and a big, hard-looking character. They stayed in the car all day waiting for him to finish work. After a few days I could not contain myself any longer, and asked what the hell they were doing there. He said they were his girlfriend and his minder, and for the twelve months he worked there, they were also there.

One night about 1am there was a knock on our door. When I answered it, there was our driver, complete with minder and girlfriend. He said, 'Can you change some silver for me?' and when I said I might have some notes and how much did he want, he produced a suitcase full of half crowns. I don't know where he got them from and I didn't want to know. He'd obviously done well somewhere, as the last time he came to see us he was living in Jersey in the Channel Islands.

On the building side about this time, Bromsgrove Council released some land on the side of a hill near Rubery, for self build. A young couple, who had tried to buy one of the houses we had built, asked if we could design and build one for them. We were lucky to find an architect called Keith Sprayson, who had a lot of flair. He designed a split level house to blend into the hillside, which was unusual then. It was a success and brought in more inquires. My brother and I were now acting as developers and as we were working, we sub-contracted the building work. We found a builder named David Keen, who built the houses for us.

Our next venture was in Halesowen. We purchased some land for six houses on another awkward site. The problem with the site was that the land was eight foot below the road. However, Keith was equal to the challenge. He designed a split level house with a bridge leading from the road to the garage and front door. There was a large family room and utility under the garage, and rooms off each half-flight of stairs. The houses were so impressive that Keith bought one for himself.

Nineteen sixty-six was drawing to a close and I was feeling more unsettled. Then, early in 1967, we saw an advert: building firm for sale. I talked David into going to have a look at it. We asked Brian Jones, our accountant, to make an appointment and we went to have a look. It was a firm called Alcester Builders and had been in existence since 1864. It had been quite a large firm in the past, but was very run down now. We decided to buy it. I would leave full-time employment to run it, and David would come when the business had improved enough to pay its way. Alcester Builders had one big thing going for it: it had a reputation second to none. I was now forty years old and had been at the Austin for 24 years. I just missed my gold watch by a few months, so my work mates bought me a gold watch as a leaving present.

From time to time people would come to assess Ian's capabilities, but they never told us anything we didn't know. In fact, they usually wasted our time and their own. Once someone came to try and talk to Ian. When we got the letter telling us the results of the assessment, it said that, since Ian was mentally handicapped, he would not be allowed to hold a driving licence. If that is not a waste of resources, tell me what is.

Meanwhile, Ian was still insisting on a rigid pattern to life, such as the ritual of shutting all the doors and locking the back door. This he referred to as 'keeping the outside out'. If we did not do this the same way every time, we had to repeat it until we got it right. At the time it was a pain in the backside but, looking back, we wonder what was going through his mind. Could we have helped him more, or was it all an inherent pattern of autism? I guess he must have felt very insecure, poor lad.

It's a wonderful thing, the human mind, when you stop to consider it. We get a problem and we just learn to live with it and work around it. When you have time to reflect, it makes you realise how much better off you are than so many other people. The one thing that has always moved me is how, when you tell someone your troubles, they confide in you too. The person you think has it all often turns out to have more problems than you. If you talk about your problems, people feel they can trust you with theirs. Mind you, there is always someone who thinks they are hard done by, while you would give your eye teeth to swap your problems for theirs.

Nineteen sixty-seven was a major turning point in our lives. I was starting a new career and Roy was changing schools. Julie was three and still travel sick, so Mom was looking after her while Margaret took Roy and Ian to school. This was still as much of a problem as ever. I had to leave home just after 6.30am to get to Alcester by 7.20 so I could open the yard and get the men off to work by 7.30. This left Margaret to manage on her own.

There were 14 men still working there. I had jumped in at the deep end, as I had to find work for them all. I had to organise all the work, go out and look at jobs, and price them. I had a lot of help there at first from the foreman, Jim Handy. He had started his apprenticeship with the firm in the 1930s, as had all the tradesmen. Jim used to look at the jobs with me and tell me how long it would take to do the work. I would add the price of the materials and arrive at a net cost. From this I would arrive at a tender figure for the job. It seemed to work OK, and things went well.

In September, Roy started at Cobham House Junior School. His headmistress at Whitford Hall thought he was too sensitive to go to such a big school, but he seemed to settle OK. We had to buy most of his quite extensive uniform at the second hand sale they held at the school. Boys seem to grow out of their clothes at an alarming rate. We got locked into private education by accident. We had sent Roy to Whitford Hall to mix with normal children and stop him copying Ian, but his progress so impressed us that we decided to stay in the private sector. Not that we could afford it at first, it was always a bit of a struggle.

I soon found myself having to go in to work on Saturdays as business picked up. Most of the men were glad of the overtime as a building labourer's take-home pay was less than £15 a week for 45 hours. This sticks in my mind, as I used to sign forms confirming it so the men could get a reduction on their rent and rates. David was still working at the Austin Motor Company; we decided he would join me at Alcester Builders early in 1968 if things were still going well enough. Anyway, he had his hands full during the latter part of 1967. He became a father when his wife Carol gave birth to twins, Steven and John, in October.

We were not able to go on holiday during 1967 as I was too far too busy at Alcester and we were hard up anyway. Ian was still very difficult, though he was starting to show signs of slowing down. It was only many years later that we realised it was his anti-convulsant drugs that were slowing him down. He still enjoyed his music, and the other thing he enjoyed was sitting in the rocking chair, so long as someone rocked him. He would also rock from side to side on his feet for hours if you did not distract him.

We kept Stafford Bull Terriers all our married life, so Ian had got used to dogs, though he never liked them. If our dog went near him, he would say, 'Ian don't like dog.' But he never hit out at the dog, and he would not object if our cat Monty sat on his lap. He never held or cuddled the cat, just let him sit there.

With Ian requiring so much of Margaret's time, we were lucky that Roy could amuse himself. He always found things to do. He was now eight and Julie was three, so while he amused himself he was also amusing Julie - at least some of the time. Mind, she did get on his nerves sometimes. We remember the time he came in from the garden with Julie screaming at him. I can't remember what they had fallen out about, but Roy simply said, 'This child needs treatment.' I suppose growing up with Ian had made him quite tolerant.

Both Roy and Julie were always very good with Ian and never seemed to resent the attention he required. Other children seemed to accept Ian better than most adults. A family named Young moved in next door, and they had four children about the same age as ours. They always asked if Ian would like to go out and play when they called for Roy. He was not capable of playing with other children, but he did like to watch them sometimes. Lea Castle, where Ian was going to school every day, only served to occupy him and did not manage to teach him anything. It would have been nice if they could have taught him to use a knife and fork, and other social skills. We were very grateful for the help they gave us, but had it have been 25 years later, with the changes that occurred in that time, they would have got a lot further with him.

Lea Castle was a large hospital with mentally handicapped people of all ages, from babies to adults. It was quite large, consisting of several buildings with four bedrooms each, a dining room and a lounge. Each bedroom had eight beds. All the buildings were in grassed areas with nice gardens, and they had named all the wards after plants and shrubs. The ones for children had names like Crocus and Primrose. The ones for older residents had names like Laurel. I think there were about 15 or 20 buildings in about 70 acres. They also had a medical centre and administration buildings. It's all different now; they have demolished most of the large units, and built bungalows to house a lot fewer residents. They have done this as part of the 'care in the community' programme, whereby the authorities move a lot of mentally ill residents into the community. This, in my opinion, is just a cost cutting exercise. It should have had much better funding to make it more effective. It was a wonderful idea that withered on the vine through lack of resources.

So Christmas was on us again, another year had gone. We finished work on Christmas Eve and went back on 2 January. Most of the men were on call for any emergency, which meant I had to be the first out to get the men, as none of them had telephones in those days.

CHAPTER FIVE

December and January were a busy time for us as Margaret's birthday was on 8 December, Ian's on the 15th, then Christmas. Mom's birthday was on 31 December, with Roy's following on 9 January. We then had a short break before Julie's birthday on 14 March. There must have been something in the air to make the sap rise in the early spring in our family!

At the start of 1968 we decided that things were now going well enough at Alcester Builders for David to leave his job and join me there full-time. He was to run the office and I would concentrate on the building work. This worked rather well, as when David started at Alcester Builders I still left home early to open the yard and give the men their work for the day. David started later, and as he had to go through Bromsgrove he was able to take Roy to school on his way to work. This was a big help to Margaret, as Roy had to be at school for 8.30am, earlier than Ian and Julie.

It was about March that we received a letter from Lea Castle Hospital, saying that some parents would now get a report rather like those from normal schools. Shortly afterwards we received a report from Mrs Sarah Sandow, Ian's class teacher. It read as follows:

Lea Castle Hospital School
Progress Report.

Name: Ian Wilkes   *D.o.b. 15.12.57.*

Although Ian has slowed down a lot lately and is not as

31

active as he has been, he clearly enjoys school and is deeply distressed if, for some reason, he cannot attend. He shows interest in peg boards and enjoys painting and drawing. I hope to increase his speed at working with pegs and screwing toys, in order to increase his chances of future employment in the workshop. He is more stable than he has been, but has outbursts of hysterical laughing and falling about which are difficult to control.

He is less antagonistic and aggressive towards the other children and will join in group activities with pleasure, particularly physical education, music and singing.

I feel that although the progress he has made is slight, he is capable of making further progress

Sarah Sandow

Ian's achievements are rather uneven. In the two sections of Communication and Occupation, he is average considering his mental handicap and age. On the other hand, there is backwardness in the Self-Help and Socialisation areas, though most of the skills required for 'scoring' are well within his ability.

H C Gunzburg, Director of Psychological Services

This was the first report we received from Ian's school. I think we did get one other but I am unable to find it. It was, of course, very different from Roy's and Julie's but we were just as proud of his progress.

Dr Patterson, who had been our only glimmer of light when Ian was at his worst, and had been so kind, had now retired. So it was with some anxiety that we waited to see what Dr Simons, who was to replace him, would be like. We worried in vain, as Dr Simons proved to be every bit as kind and helpful as Dr Patterson over the years to follow. We decided to try to go on holiday later in the summer so we booked a holiday at Butlins in Minehead. Ever the optimists, we thought Ian would enjoy all the activity.

We arrived Saturday lunchtime, booked in and explained Ian's problems to the reception staff. They were very kind and said, 'Don't worry, if he plays up we'll understand.' You cannot overestimate how support like this bolsters you up, especially after most people's reactions. Mind you, I think there is much more tolerance today.

Ian was very unhappy all that first day, and played up during dinner, which was most unlike him as he liked his food. Things didn't get any better that evening and he even played up during the night. So in the morning we decided the only thing to do was for me to take him home, while Margaret stayed for the rest of the week to give Julie and Roy a holiday. When I started the car Ian seemed to know we were going home as he settled down and was as good as gold all the way home. Julie and Roy had a lovely holiday and Margaret had a well-deserved break. Ian was quite good and when we went back to collect the family he behaved well. After this episode we decided to ask if Ian could stay at Lea Castle if we went on holiday the next year. They said they would have him.

Later that summer I took Julie to London for a few days' holiday, thinking that we could visit the museums and see some of the sights. But Julie wanted to spend most of the time in Trafalgar Square, feeding the pigeons! So that had to be the first and last stop every day. I had to bribe her to visit other places by promising to take her to the pictures every evening. A good job we were only stopping three nights, which is plenty in a large city. London is a lovely place to visit, in small doses.

Back at work things were starting to buzz. Work was coming in fast and we were growing fast. We had to employ a surveyor to make sure we were getting paid for all the work we were doing on the larger jobs. I spent more time with the men on site than in the office, so I got to know them quite well. Some of the stories they told about how hard the work was in the 1930s were hair-raising, although in the 1960s it was still labour intensive. For example, when a load of bricks came on site, we had to unload them by hand (there were up to 10 000 bricks in a load), usually with all the men standing in a line about five foot apart and throwing them from one to the next in line, about five bricks at a time. Everyone had to join in, and if I was on site the shout was 'Come on, get in line, gaffer' - and no gloves either. It was worse in the winter as a lot of bricklayers had cracked and bleeding hands, due to the cement and cold weather.

I was in the joiner's shop one day talking to Jim Handy, who was telling me about life in the building trade before the war. He said that he had been an apprentice for about a year in 1936. One day, one of the brothers who owned the business came up to him and asked him how long he'd been there. Jim said, 'Twelve months, Mr Buggins.' Harry Buggins said, 'Well, you're old enough now. I've got a pauper to bury up at the workhouse, and as I only get two pounds ten shillings it's an apprentice's job. I can't afford to send a tradesman. So go up to the workhouse, see the superintendent and he'll show you the body. Measure it up, come back to the yard, sort out enough timber from the scrap pile at the bottom of the yard to make a coffin. Then put it on the hand cart, take it up to the workhouse and someone will help you put the body in the box. When the labourer has dug the grave, let the curate know and take the body up to the church for him.' Such was an apprentice's lot in the 1930s.

By 1969 we were into a routine and time was flying. At home Ian was quieter, but still seemed prone to aggressive outbursts. At one time Margaret's legs were black and blue where he had kicked her. When we told them at Lea Castle, they merely asked what we did when he kicked out. Margaret said, 'Get out of the way if I can.' They found that funny but didn't have much advice to offer. When Ian was in an aggressive mood it was a wonder that Roy and Julie did not come to some harm. We never did find out what started his outbursts. Although they occurred less frequently in later years, he was subject to them all his life.

We decided to give the holidays a miss that year but Roy had the chance to go to camp with the cub scouts. They were going to the Lake District, to a lovely spot alongside a lake. They had a lot of fun that week. It's such a shame that so few people give up their time to run these organisations today. In no time it was back to the old routine: taking the children to school. The busier you are the faster the time seems to go. No sooner were we over the summer holidays than Christmas was on us again. Either my memory is fading, or nothing out of the ordinary happened in 1969.

Nineteen seventy was another year of change, for during my travels round the jobs I saw a house for sale in Stock Green near Inkberrow. I had a look around it. It was a total wreck, the sort of challenge I liked. I took Margaret to see it and she said, 'I'm not moving in there until you've finished it'. We made an offer and started work sometime in March. The house had quite a history. It was a half timbered house built originally on common land. The frame had been made up in the forest and carried to the site. Then all the family and friends would have gathered early one morning to erect it and build the hearth and chimney. Anyone could build a house on common land, but you had to have the roof on and a fire lit within 24 hours. The only way we were able to date the building was from the style of the numbers on all the joints - they put the date of construction between the 15th and 16th centuries. Builders in those days had to number the joints so they could erect the house on site. They had to dismantle it to carry it to the site; there were no cranes in those days.

In 1857, Parliament appointed 'two gentlemen of Oxford to apportion and appoint the waste and common lands of Inkberrow, Stock and Bradley'. They sold these plots off by public auction at the Swan Inn at Alcester Warwickshire. Old Crown Cottage sold with four acres, and the man who bought it applied for a liquor license - hence its name, the Old Crown Inn. I wonder where all the cash from the sale went. I would take a bet that the poor devils they ejected from their homes never got a penny. People were being turned off their land in England, Wales, as well as Scotland and Ireland in those days. It was common land belonging to the people. Tens of thousands of acres were stolen from the common people in England and Wales during the 18th and 19th centuries, while in Scotland and Ireland the people thrown off their lands were tenants.

When we started work on the Old Crown Cottage, I had some of my employees doing the work at weekends. One was Reg

Hands, a bricklayer in his late sixties. After his first day's work Reg found that he was covered in fleas when he got home. His wife made him strip off in the back garden and hosed him down before letting him into the house. This continued for the next six weekends until all the fleas were gone.

That spring Roy took the exam to go to the senior school. He was awarded a scholarship, which was a huge help to us financially.

Later that summer I thought that we could all do with a break; my working seven days a week threw a lot on Margaret's shoulders, so we needed it. We booked a holiday cottage in Fishguard in Wales, so we could try taking Ian on holiday again. The cottage was a disaster, as it was filthy. It was an old British Rail cottage in the middle of hundreds of others. I wanted to turn around and come home, but Margaret insisted on staying and spent the first two days scrubbing the place out so we could have our holiday. We were luckily that Ian seemed to settle OK and enjoyed his days on the beach. We travelled down as far as St David's and found some lovely beaches; the only problem was that Margaret got her legs badly sunburnt and kept fainting. I don't think we had heard of sun block in those days - you either covered up or suffered.

September came and Roy started at the senior school, He started school at 8.30am and as they had to do their prep at school, he didn't finish till 8pm. One of us had to go and collect him every night, and as he had to go six days a week, plus Sunday morning, it meant a lot of running about. Ian always came too, and he must have known where he was because if you headed toward Kidderminster he would get upset.

A big change was in store for Ian, at least from his point of view as he liked a rigid routine. In mid-September we had a letter from Ian's teacher, saying that she was leaving at the end of the month, as her husband had got a new job and they had to move to Hull. In her letter she said.:

I shall be sorry to leave Lea Castle in many ways, not least because I shall have to stop teaching Ian, whom I have known for such a long time. Of course just lately he hasn't been very active in the classroom, but when he is able and willing to join in, he really enjoys himself. I think he is a much nicer and friendlier person than he was when I first knew him five years ago. I hope he will be very happy with the new arrangements for him. I have been very glad to know you both as well as the children, and am very grateful for all the sweets biscuits, and squash you have brought for the class over the years. I do hope to see you before I go.

Sarah Sandow.

Although Ian was so difficult most of the time, everyone who had contact with him over a period of time was genuinely fond of him. The sad thing was that Ian's behaviour frightened off a lot of people. The severity of his fits even seemed to frighten people who had some experience of epilepsy. This was one of the reason why we could never get anyone to look after Ian while we had a night out, to let off steam.

After our holiday we had to think about selling the bungalow and getting ready to move. The estate agents said that the motorway being so close by would reduce the price of the bungalow quite considerably, and even then it took a long time to sell. We were finally able to move into Old Crown Cottage shortly before Christmas 1970. We still had a building site to turn into a garden, but by now we were getting used to that.

CHAPTER SIX

Old Crown Cottage was a much larger house than anything we had lived in before, and it backed on to woodland. We were quite unused to the silence after living next to the motorway for so long; but you get used to silence much quicker than you adapt to the noise of traffic when they build a motorway along your garden. We soon settled in and had our first Christmas on our own in years. It made a lovely change. Julie and Roy had big bedrooms and Ian had his room adjoining our bedroom so we could hear him when he started to fit. Ian would have a *grand mal* fit in the night once or twice a week. When you have a child like Ian you seem to sleep with one ear open, waiting for his next fit. When it happened we would dash in to him and lay him on his side in the recovery position. Ian became very distressed after having a fit, not knowing where he was, so we liked to be there to comfort him.

As we got into the early part of 1971 we had our first experience of Ian going into status, which is when someone has one fit after another without recovering in between. Having no experience and not having been advised what to do if this happened, I panicked. I got my car (an estate), dropped the seats down, carried Ian down to the car and laid him in the back. We got Roy and Julie in as well and made a dash to Lea Castle about 20 miles away. When we arrived at 2.30am, we roused the night staff, who put Ian on oxygen and gave him an injection of vellum. After they got him a bed in a ward, the nurse in charge came out and gave us a real telling off. She said we could have killed him by moving him around. In future, she said, call your GP out to give him an injection.

So when it happened again a few weeks later, Dr Pinnock from Astwood Bank came out at about 4am. He was always fantastic with Ian, and never complained about being got out of bed in the middle of the night. He injected the drug directly into the muscle, so it was very painful and Ian would scream in agony, which was most upsetting. Sometimes the doctor would send for the ambulance to take Ian to the hospital in Worcester for observation. Although Ian was very difficult, he always seemed to be the nurses' favourite and they always made a fuss of him.

One night in June the birds were singing so loud that it woke us all up. We could not think what it was, then the penny dropped: nightingales singing. So we got Julie and Roy out of bed to listen to them. We were up for over an hour that first night, and they sang so loudly it was unbelievable. After a few nights you come to accept it, although Roy did go out after midnight one night to record the nightingales on a small reel-to-reel tape recorder. We had it for many years, and it was so clear when we played it back.

In the back garden I built a swing out of scaffolding tube and concreted it into the ground. It was one of the few things that Ian liked, as long as you pushed him. He spent hours on it, which also had the advantage of amusing Roy and Julie. The next door neighbour, however, complained that Roy could see them when they were in their garden, (over the six foot fence) and would he please stop. I could not repeat my comments here. We did get friendly with Les Harrison who lived on a small holding opposite our house. Les still comes to see us nearly every week, even after all these years.

We had another shock waiting in the wings. My mother had to go to the hospital to see a specialist as her doctor said she had breast cancer. My sister Margot and I went with her. The specialist had a weird bedside manner; as Mom came out of the examination room he said, 'You are a very foolish woman, you know you are going to die, don't you?' I think this was because she had left it too late, and had been going to a faith healer for quite long time. She always had a horror of hospitals. That summer she had a lot of chemotherapy, but all it did was delay the inevitable for a short time.

Early that year we had booked a holiday at Pontins in the Isle of Wight, so we decided to carry on and take the children away. We had arranged for Ian to stay at Lea Castle for the week. We all had a wonderful time going around the island to see the sights, as well as taking advantage of the in-camp entertainment. Julie was Princess Pontin for the week. She did not like it when the boy who was Prince for the week had to kiss her. Roy won the Donkey Derby, so they both had a prize. A couple of mornings Julie and I went horse riding, which was when she caught the bug for horses. She had to wait till the next year before she had her first pony.

After we got back and collected Ian, we found he was still going into status, and it was always at night. So we made arrangements to see his specialist at Lea Castle. After looking at Ian's records he said he would change his drugs. Ian was to come off his Phenobarbitone and be put on Epilim. He had been on Phenobarbitone for so long that, as it was addictive, he would have to go into hospital to be weaned off it. The specialist arranged for Ian to go to Lea Castle for six weeks. We found out many years later that they should have taken 12 months to withdraw his Phenobarbitone. The staff said we should not visit him during this time as it would upset him too much. This was a bad mistake, because when we fetched him home he had lost a lot of weight and was all hollow-chested. He could not hold a cup to drink out of as he was shaking so much, and we had to feed him as well as help him drink. God only knows what he went through, poor lamb. It was like someone addicted to heroin going cold turkey.

It was about two months before he had recovered enough to go back to school at Lea Castle. They then informed us that he was too old to go there, as they only took them up to 14, and he would have to go into the workshop. After the workshop tried him for a couple of weeks, they said he was not capable of doing any work. They also said he would have to stay on one of the wards, and suggested he should stay overnight during the week. After much soul-searching we decided to give it a try, so we started by taking him on Monday morning and collecting him Friday afternoon. He got so upset on Monday and so happy on Friday that it soon became Tuesday and Thursday. That was soon to change when Mom came to stay for Christmas. When she first came she seemed so much brighter but after Christmas she went downhill fast. With Margaret looking after Mom, Ian had to stay full-time at Lea Castle. It was heartbreaking when we went to visit him on the weekends; he wanted so much to come home with us, but we thought it was for the best.

We were into 1972 and Mom was fading fast, and in a lot of pain. Dr Pinnock was fantastic with Mom as he came in every night between 9 and 11pm to give her a morphine injection, and the nurse came every morning. By the time we got into February Mom was much worse and was soon in bed all the time. A lot of relatives came to see her from time to time.

One strange thing did happen while she was quite lucid. She would often ask Julie who her little friend was, when Julie had no one with her. Mom would describe the 'friend', including the way she was dressed. We were to find out much later that a young girl had died in the cottage and they had buried her in the garden.

As we came towards the end of February Mom was sedated all the time, and Margaret was sitting up with her every night. On the evening of the 26 February, when Dr Pinnock came to give her the evening injection, he said, 'I don't think she will last the night'. That night Tony, Margot's husband, said he would stop up with Margaret. I left them to it and went to bed in the early hours of 27 February. Then another strange thing happened. I seemed to wake in the night reaching for Margaret. I remember saying, 'Help me, I'm dying.' Then I had a very funny sensation, like a whirlpool starting in my stomach and going up through my head. Then I was looking down on myself lying in bed. The feeling of total peace and comfort was unbelievable. Afterwards I sat up in bed feeling so relaxed that I felt had to tell Margaret about it.

At about 5am I went into Mom's bedroom. Margaret and Tony were sitting with her, and said that there was no change. So I told them about my experience, and said that if this was how it was when you died there was nothing to be afraid of. I then said I would go and make a cup of tea, and as I went down the stairs to the kitchen. Margaret called me and said that Mom had sat up in bed and as she fell back she died. It was as if she had been afraid to let go, until I said how peaceful it was on the other side. We rang the doctor, who came and issued the death certificate. He also examined Margaret's legs, which had become badly swollen. He told her to go to bed and stay there till the funeral, as she had not been to bed for over two weeks through stopping up with my mom.

But Margaret, being Margaret, was up and about getting the housework done the next day. We fetched Ian home for Mom's funeral, and decided to take Ian to Lea castle on Tuesdays and bring him home on Thursdays again. We had found out that all Ian was doing was sitting around on the ward with no stimulation. So we decided that he would only stay away for two nights, to give him a change of scenery. The hospital staff could monitor his fits. They were very good, but they were working under many difficulties. There were not enough staff to occupy the residents, and all their time was taken up feeding and attending to the patients' personal needs. With only one or two staff on duty overnight, it was hard work for them. There was a single supervisor who went round the wards during the night, who was also on call in any emergency. So all of the time that we were taking Ian to stay overnight we were worrying if we were doing the right thing.

At work things were still going well, and we were getting some nice jobs, like constructing the new library in Pershore for Worcestershire County Council. The architect was from the London area, and when I set the building out it was too big to fit into the gap between the existing buildings. When I rang him he said was I using a rubber tape. So I told him the county clerk of works was signing daywork sheets for the men and machines on site until he sorted it out. He was on site within four hours. When he checked it and said I was right, I asked him if he used a rubber tape when he did the original design. He had the cheek to say that he never checked it before he designed the building, only used the county maps.

On the small works side we were doing a lot of maintenance, all on daywork, which included work on Warwickshire County Council schools, fire stations, police stations, courts and assorted houses. The supervision for the work was done by the clerk of works for Warwickshire County Council, Walter Roberts, who was an ex-tradesman. So he knew what he was doing, which made a change from a lot of the college-trained men they seemed to employ.

We were also doing the maintenance on a lot of National Trust property: Packwood house, Coughton Court, Hanbury Hall, and all the farms and other properties they own. In addition, we were maintaining the canal from Stratford to the Grand Union junction at Lapworth. Major Grundy was responsible for the canal, as well as Packwood House and would ask for five or six men from October to Easter. They were all on daywork and he would tell the men where he wanted them to go, and what he wanted doing. The buildings maintenance was the responsibility of Mr Goadsby, the building manager from the area office in Tewkesbury. He was very good, knew what he wanted and expected it to be right. As an ex-tradesman and site agent, he also knew all about the job. We were also doing a lot of the restoration work at Ragley Hall. It's quite an eye-opener when you see behind the scenes in a stately home. From the way the servants had to live and the rooms they lived in, you can imagine what a life of drudgery a lot of them had.

During the summer of 1972 we decided to look for a pony for Julie, and when I mentioned it at work one of the joiners, Eric Blundell, said he had one to sell. His daughter had outgrown it, so we did a deal. When we'd rebuilt the house the garage had been a stable before we converted it, so I had to convert it back again. The pony was called Crackers (his name, not his nature, as he was cream coloured: cream crackers, get it?) We now had to learn some animal husbandry, not only how to look after the pony but also what illnesses to look out for, what kind of straw he needed for bedding, what hay, how many nuts he'd eat and so on. Crackers soon settled into his new home, but our next problem was finding some pasture for him.

That year we went to Pontins Barton Hall for our holidays. Like most people, a week was the best we could do. Luckily we all had a lovely time, as it was to be our last holiday together for some years.

After we got back, Lady Isabel from Coughton Court asked me to convert her stable block into an art gallery. We did this and one day Margaret and I received an invitation to the grand opening. We put on our Sunday best and when we arrived the butler handed us a glass of champagne. While I was walking around, a very large cut-glass bowl on a stem caught my eye. Being nosy by nature, I picked it up and turned it over to see if the price was underneath. Little did I realise that the top was separate from the bottom, and it dropped onto the flagstone floor, which was covered by a thin hessian carpet. I caught it on the first bounce, undamaged. I then thought I would have to catch Margaret as she'd gone all weak at the knees, wondering if we would have to take out another mortgage to pay for it. One of the assistants came up and said in a snooty voice, 'Is everything all right?' I said, 'Fine now.' I'd never felt such fear and such relief within such a short space of time!

A little later in the year, while we were doing some work on the court, I saw Lady Isabel unloading some paintings from her car. She said, 'How do you like these?' I looked through them and said that I liked a set of four watercolours. When I told her I liked them she said, 'I got them at a bargain price so you can have them for what I paid for them.' When she told me the price I said I only wanted two of them; it was all I could afford. The price I paid for them was £19 and £16. Not long afterwards, I had a call from someone who had bought the other two paintings. He offered me £150 for the two I had. I must admit that it was a temptation but Margaret said, 'If you like them, keep them.' I am glad we did now, as we had them valued in 1990 and were told they were worth £1000 each. That was a lucky day when I saw them being unloaded from Lady Isabel's car.

CHAPTER SEVEN

A s Christmas approached we started to look for some property with land. It was hard to find anywhere at a price we could afford, so we decided to leave it till the Spring. Roy was doing very well now at school. The school had moved him up a class, which meant he would take his 'O' levels at 15 instead of 16. He was also a good athlete. He ran for the school, was in the first team for rugby and cricket, and also ran for the county. Julie, too, was enjoying school and doing well.

Ian was still spending some time every week at Lea Castle, but not getting much benefit from it. He really needed more stimulation, but we were at a loss about what to do. So time just drifted on, and Ian grew more withdrawn. Margaret did her best to occupy him when he was home. She would sing nursery rhymes to him while pushing him on the swing. Ian loved this but put his own words to them. Strangely enough, he always got the tune correct.

My Aunt Dora was very fond of Ian and would chatter away to him when we went to see her in Leamington Spa. She always fascinated him. He would sit dumbstruck when we were there, and not say a word. At home, when singing his nursery rhymes, he would use phrases like 'Aunt Dora talk', 'Margot goes to the pictures', 'Mummy swears', 'Don't like dogs' and 'cup of tea shop'. He could fit them all together so it sounded quite musical. When he was happy that the rhyme was right, he would shout with excitement He also liked catching a ball, having his hair combed, and especially having a bath. He was now responding more to personal contact, although he still showed a lot of his other autistic tendencies, such as rocking and getting upset if things were not done to a strict routine. He also still had obsessions with some words. If you said the wrong word, in whatever context, he would jump up and down, squeal and shout, 'Daddy, don't say dog!' or whatever. This could be most disconcerting, especially if you were talking to a stranger who didn't know Ian.

Margaret was still running back and forth to Bromsgrove, driving Roy and Julie to and from school. She also had to look after a big house and amuse Ian when he was home, which left little time for any social life. We did, however, have our moments. Every year there was a charity ball at Ragley Hall, and that year we went with three other couples. The tickets were £15 per couple. They had a ten-piece band playing in the great hall. It started at 10pm and went on till 4am. The champagne was free, with waitresses filling your glass every time you went to dance. After midnight you went downstairs for a buffet meal: all the meats and trimmings you could think of, with a lovely selection of sweets. At about 4am they auctioned the flowers off; I was so drunk that I paid £27 for a small bunch of flowers. Brian Jones, our accountant, took my car keys off me and gave them to Margaret, telling her she'd have to drive. They helped me into the car and when Margaret got home, she came round and opened my door. I promptly fell out on to the gravel drive. Every ten minutes or so she came out of the house, gave me a kick and said, 'Lionel, get up and come in or the rats will bite you.' After about an hour I crawled into the house on my knees and Margaret managed to roll me onto the settee. I slept for a couple of hours and woke up feeling as if I had slept all night. I have heard that if you get drunk on champagne it doesn't leave you with a headache, and this experience seemed to prove that right.

Talking of rats, it was about this time that we noticed a terrible smell every time we went into the dining room. After a while you became used to it, so it was very difficult to locate where it was coming from. So I sent Reg Ainge, one of the small works crew, to find it. The ceiling had beams with plaster board in between them.

Reg cut a hole in each one in turn, and smelt the hole. At the fifth one there was a loud shout, and when Reg cut the panel out we found the body of the biggest rat I have ever seen. Earlier we had found a hole big enough to put your fist through the wall behind Roy's bedside cupboard. The rat had also made a hole in the cupboard where Roy had a habit of hoarding his sweets, which had attracted our king rat. After that he had to keep his sweets in a tin box in another part of his bedroom.

Back at work we were employing more men. One of these was a labourer named Martin. He was not very bright but was the strongest lad I have ever met, and I was in a weightlifting team when I first got married. Martin had never had a proper meal in his life, as his parents spent all their time in pubs. He had spent most of his childhood on pub doorsteps, because in those days they did not allow children to go in pubs. One day a ten-ton load of cement came into the yard and Martin was one of the men who unloaded it. When cement came direct from the factory it was red hot, and all the men put coats on to carry the bags into the store. As it was a very hot day, Martin would not put his coat on and consequently burned his shoulders. A few days later I asked Bert Coles the lorry driver to take some materials to a site, which included ten cwts of cement. So Bert told Martin to start loading the cement while he came into the office to get the details. When we came out Martin was carrying two bags at a time, holding them on his arms in front of him away from his body as if they were still hot, although they were now quite cold. I would not have believed anybody could have done it.

One of the reps who came to the office from time to time demonstrated a new device for clearing drains. It was a pump-up piece of equipment that sent a shock wave through the water to the blockage and cleared it. It impressed me so much that I purchased one. It went into the stores but it appeared that no one wanted to use it. Then one day we had a blockage just up the high street, and I was in the yard when Bert Coles and Fred Rose came in to get more rods. When I asked them how it was going, they said they could not reach the blockage and would have to dig up

47

part of the drain. I asked if they'd tried the new pump. 'Not likely!' was the reply I got. So I said I would bloody well show them how to do it then. We got the box containing all the bits and pieces that went with it, and off we went to clear the drain. As I was just off to a site meeting, dressed in a suit and tie instead of my usual work clothes, I should have known better.

When we got there they were still reluctant to use it, so I said, 'Pump it up and I'll do it.' While they were pumping it up I assembled the pipes to go into the sewer. I was in such a hurry that I forgot a most important part; I didn't put the plug on the pipe. I inserted the pipe down the drain and fired the pump. After a second or two the sewage in the manhole went down with a gurgle and I turned to Bert and Fred and said, 'There you are, easy isn't it?' I saw them jump back but before I could ask what was the matter the sewage came roaring back up the manhole and drenched me. All I could think to say was, 'You'd better get the pick and shovel and start digging.' When I walked down the High Street with my jacket in one hand and socks and shoes in the other, for some reason everyone gave me a wide berth. When I got back to the yard, half the people we employed seemed to have heard about it, and were there to cheer me. I never did live it down.

Our bull terrier dogs would never go upstairs in the Old Crown Cottage. You could not drag them up, but one day when Margaret was in the kitchen, she heard an unearthly scream coming from the first floor. As she raced upstairs to see what it was, the dogs got there first but there was nothing in sight. A few days later she saw the figure of a young girl coming down the stairs and as she got to the bottom she vanished. We think it must have been the same girl my mother had seen. The dogs on this occasion just disappeared and didn't show their faces for some time. They got upset several times during our time at Stock Green, but we never saw anything again. I think that dogs are much more sensitive to strange happenings than most people.

We didn't have a holiday in 1973 as we had found a place in Bishampton called Ivy House Farm. It had all the farm buildings and six and a half acres of land, with planning permission for a new house to one side of the farm house. The price was £30 000. We put the cottage up for sale, and within days the agent told us he had a sale at the asking price. As the amount of interest shown was intense, I told him I felt that we should ask for sealed bids by a certain date. This upset the estate agent, and he tried to get us to accept the, £18 000 he had set the price at. We had the feeling that the person he wanted to have it was a friend of his. Two weeks later we opened the tenders and the best one was £23 850, so it was worth holding out.

We waited for the summer school holidays before we moved so we would not have the problem of taking the children to school while moving. In some ways we felt quite sad leaving Stock Green, as we had so many memories associated with the cottage, although we were only there a short time. I often wonder if anyone else has had any odd experiences there. Some houses just have an atmosphere. You can feel at ease in some and on edge in others. Margaret always liked Old Crown Cottage and often said she wished she could move it, to wherever we were living at the time.

Ian was 16, Roy 14 and Julie nine when we made the move to Bishampton. So this would mean Margaret travelling more miles to take the children to school and Ian to Kidderminster, as Bishampton was a few miles further from Bromsgrove than Stock Green. So another moving day finally arrived, and on a lovely day we set off to our new home.

CHAPTER EIGHT

We arrived at Ivy House Farm, late July 1973. We had left Ian at Lea Castle for two extra days so we could move in without upsetting him. The day we moved in, Rusty our Staffordshire bull terrier went exploring, which resulted in us being introduced to our new neighbours, Robin and Shirley Lloyd. Rusty had gone through the hedge to next door. Robin was lying under a car repairing it (his house was also the local garage and blacksmiths). Rusty cocked his leg over Robin's backside and soaked it. Robin swore and tried to jump up, forgetting he was under the car. He cut his head just as I arrived looking for Rusty. It seemed a fine time to introduce myself! As I got back home I was just in time to see Robin's cat run off with our budgie. I did manage to get it off the cat, but the poor bird died the next day.

We found that we had inherited five farm cats, fifteen bantam hens with two cocks. The two bantam cockerels were beautiful, very vivid colours, but could be quite vicious when strangers went too near. They would fly at them and try to rake them with their spurs. The cats lived in the barns and they were also wild. We decided to have them neutered and consulted the vet about how we were to catch them. He gave us some drugged bait and when they passed out we put them in boxes, but by the time we got them to the vets they had come round. They were going berserk in the boxes, and I didn't envy him the task of getting them out. He was unable to neuter one as she was having kittens, so we had to wait till she had them. We soon tamed the kittens and they lived in the house with us, where the dogs quickly accepted them. Staffordshires are very gentle with any young animals or human babies, so there are no problems. Julie's pony Crackers also settled with all that grass and nice stables.

After two days we went to fetch Ian home. It was quite amazing that he took to the farmhouse straight away. He insisted that he was not a cottage boy, he was a farm boy. This pleased us, because we'd been worried that he would miss the cottage. It became obvious that the important thing in Ian's life was being with his family, although he still went stiff if you tried to hug him.

Shortly after our move, we decided that, since Ian was getting no benefit from going to Lea Castle, we would have him at home full-time. They tried to talk us out of it, but it had been worrying us for some time. So home he came to stay. There was plenty to occupy him around the farm, but of course most of this fell on Margaret's head. We soon got very friendly with some of our neighbours, particularly Robin and Shirley Lloyd and Robin's business partner Bill Tredwell. Bill was interested in all farm animals, and he had been a farrier many years ago, so he was a lot of help with Crackers. Bill lived with Robin's granny, Mrs Lloyd, and they had some land where Bill kept some sheep and cattle

It was not long before Bill told us that he knew someone who wanted to sell a Jersey cow that was in milk, so I was soon learning to milk. When you first sit on a three-legged stool with your face against the side of a cow, it is magic. Then reality soon intrudes when she lifts her tail and shits all over the floor. A cow is a big animal so there is quite a lot of it. Inevitably some of it runs down her tail and it's not too long before she lashes out with her tail. This soon connects with your face - one of the more earthy pleasures of smallholding!

The question was: what could you do with nearly two gallons of milk a day? Obviously you make butter. Our first attempts with the Kenwood produced butter but soon it burnt out the machine. Bill came to the rescue again. He told us he had seen an old hand churn in a junk shop in Worcester, so off we went to Worcester to buy it. It was so simple, like an old glass sweet jar with a wooden paddle and a handle on top. It held over half a gallon of cream, and made the butter in five minutes. You then wash the butter, using the wooden paddles to knock the water out, and add salt if required. The next problem was how to separate the cream from the milk. I solved this by making a pin-hole in empty one-gallon plastic ice-cream containers and filling them with milk, after putting a pin in to plug the hole in the bottom of the container. Left overnight, the cream settled on the top. We then pulled the plug and out ran the skimmed milk, leaving the cream in the container. After two or three days we had enough cream to make our butter. It's amazing how quickly you get into a routine: up at 6am, do the milking and turn out the animals, then it's off to work to open the yard for 7.30. If you get up late you can't hurry the animals, so it really is a wonderful way to ease the tensions and pressures of modern living.

Ian had settled very well, but he never forgot the way to Lea Castle. If we went out and headed towards Kidderminster, you could see the tension in him. He would start saying, 'Ian's a farm boy'. But when you turned off that road, he would relax. He had some funny little ways, and he loved to tell tales. He would say to Margaret, 'Daddy swears' or 'Daddy let Polly out of prison', his polite was of telling the world when I farted. It used to make his day if anyone dropped a plate and broke it; he would laugh fit to bust. He would get excited if he heard a baby cry, not that we knew why, as he rarely cried himself, and he would say, 'Ian don't cry.' On the rare occasions he did cry we would cry with him, as he seemed so pathetic. His main pleasure in life was still going to a shop to buy a toy gun or car. He never seemed to grasp that who ever was with him was paying for it, he always thought the person serving had given it to him as a present.

We were stocking up with animals now. We had purchased two goats in milk and a piglet to fatten for bacon. We had the goats to provide milk when we dried off Daisy, our cow, before she had her calf. (All our animals had names.)

Tom Parry, who lived up the High Street and reared store cattle, came to see us a couple of months after we moved in. He asked if we would let a local girl keep her pony, a 16-hand grey called

Magic, with us. He said her father had died and the place she kept her horse had put the rent up so much she could no longer afford it, as she was still at school. Ruth was about the same age as Roy. We thought someone who was good with horses would help Julie, so that was how Ruth Barton came into our lives. She is still a good friend today. Ruth was always very good to Ian, and after she qualified as a teacher she worked at the local school for mentally handicapped and autistic children. This type of school didn't exist when Ian was young, worse luck.

Our holding was now getting stocked up. We had hens, geese and a calf to rear, which we fed on the goat's milk, as Jersey milk is too rich for any calf except their own.

I was now looking into the design for a new house we were planning to build; then we would sell the farm house. We thought that we could build the new house, sell the old and be left without a mortgage, but you never know what fate has in store. The best-laid plans of mice and men gang aft aglee, as Rabbie Burns once said. I contacted a local architect we did work for, and discussed what we wanted. But my eyes were bigger than my belly, as my granny always used to say when we asked for more than we could eat. So we ended up with the design for a lovely house, but it had a floor area of 3 000 square feet. This was about three times as big as the average three-bedroom estate house.

Over the Christmas break Roy and I started to clear the area for the new house. In January 1974 I got a couple of our men digging the footings. It was Harold Taylor and his mate Bubby who sub-contracted some of Alcester Builders' groundworks. I built the whole house ready for occupation in well under six months and never had more than three men working on it at any one time.

Opposite our house there was a little bungalow owned and occupied by an old couple, Dolly Andrews and her husband. Dolly was lovely with Ian and always made a fuss of him, in spite of him being so difficult at times. Ian seemed to respond to her, and would get quite excited when Margaret took him to see her.

With people coming and going all the time and with all the various works with the animals, Ian seemed to keep interested. Although he never had any rapport with the animals, he never showed any distress being around them and was never unkind to them. Ian was 17 now and getting to be a big lad, so he was becoming difficult to handle when he had an epileptic fit, or had a tantrum. When Ian got upset Margaret found that the answer was to distract him, but this was easier said than done. She would calm him down by doing the things that gave him pleasure, like combing his hair, rubbing his back or if that didn't work giving him a bath. He now seemed to have an obsession with the weather. He would say, 'Ian don't like rain or don't like wind' or 'Don't let sky rain'. It must have been the words themselves that he disliked, because at times he would stand out in the rain or wind rocking like mad and this was a sure sign that he was enjoying himself.

In any work with nature, such as farming, the seasons rule your life. So we had to move into the new house between hay-making and baling the straw for the animal bedding. I helped Robin and Bill with theirs and they cut and baled our hay, which saved having to pay someone to do it. Although hay-making is hard work, it's such a lot of fun when you do it together, pulling each other's legs and tapping the cider bottle. It's amazing how much strong cider you can drink and stay sober when you are sweating it out all day. It reminded me of the time I was on maintenance in foundries and stamp shops when I was an apprentice - the drinking, that is. The men operating the machines worked stripped to the waist in hot and filthy conditions, drinking six or eight pints of beer a day. Although we were working hard, at least we were out in the open air in some of the loveliest countryside in the world.

We decided that as we were only moving next door into the new house we would move ourselves. Big mistake! They say every man to his own trade. It took Roy and me three weeks of hard work to carry our furniture out of one house and across the yard into the new house. Margaret worked just as hard packing and unpacking while Julie was doing her best to help her and amuse Ian. It was a good job the move came in Roy's school holidays or I would still be there! One of the problems was I was working during the day, and of course we still had to do the milking and attend to the animals before we ate.

The next mistake we made was to hold a jumble sale in the new house in aid of the local Mencap Society. We cleared the lounge to lay out all the goods we had collected for the sale, then we advertised it. When the day finally arrived, the people came rushing in. They soon stripped the place and we found later that a lot of our small private possessions had gone too, and not been paid for. They say you should learn from your mistakes, but we never seem to.

After the school holidays, Roy decided that as he had taken his 'O' levels, he now wanted to sit his 'A' levels. But he wanted to go to one of the local schools to study for them, as he was getting tired of the long hours at Bromsgrove School. The headmaster got very annoyed when I went to tell him. He said the scholarship could have gone to someone who would have stayed to take the 'A' level exams. Margaret and I thought that if Roy was not keen on going, he would not work as hard. We got him in to Prince Henrys at Evesham, which was about to change from a grammar school to a comprehensive. He enjoyed the more relaxed atmosphere so much that before the end of the year we had a letter from the headmaster, Stanley English, saying that if Roy didn't do some work soon he would not pass any exams. But Roy proved him wrong the next year when he sailed through his 'A' levels.

During the school holidays Julie went to spend a week at a riding stable to learn how to handle her pony. She went to Mrs Bomford at Moyfield stables in South Littleton, who was and still is a wonderful riding teacher. When Julie came back we realised that Crackers was too small now and we would have to buy her a larger pony. We were about enter a very murky world. People think some car dealers are shady, but remember, horse traders have been at it a lot longer and some are very shady indeed. The trouble is that when you enter the world of horse traders for the first time, you don't know the good from the bad and of course there are both.

We had vetted the ponies we were interested in to see if they were sound in wind and limb. The one that Julie wanted was a gelding, a lovely pony of 14 hands. The vet said he was sound but that he personally would not buy him as the pony needed more schooling. But Julie wanted him and we were getting tired of looking, so we took him on and called him Star. We had a lot of fun at first trying to get someone to ride him, but it was soon a pain because Julie couldn't go out on him. So we arranged for someone to come and school him.

The trainer turned up with his 12-year old son in tow. When I realised he intended to let the boy ride Star, I said it would be too much for him. But the trainer said, 'He can ride anything', so we tacked Star up. The boy mounted him in the field, and when we let him go, Star set off across the field like something out of a western movie, bucking and twisting. The lad's riding hat came off and I got quite worried for him. However, he stayed on the horse and after some time his father said, 'We'd better take him home for a month as there's nothing we can do here'. When Star came back he was rideable but was always frisky. One day he threw Julie as she was mounting in the yard and she fell on her head; although she had her hat on she ended up in hospital with concussion. We decided that he would have to go and started the search for another pony. Julie's new pony, Katie, was a mare 14½ hands high and much more manageable.

As Ian's 18th birthday approached it made us sad, because had Ian not been handicapped, it would have been one of the highlights in his life. He would have been leaving school and starting a new phase in his life. As it was, he was still a 5-year old in a man's body. We were lucky in that Ian's sexual drive had not developed. This can cause a lot of problems in some young handicapped adults. He was still suffering from severe fits and it was a pleasure when he went two or three days without having one.

On one occasion, when we took Ian to Lea Castle to have his blood tested to check his drug levels, the nurse took the blood from his arm. The little puncture wound didn't seem to heal and it slowly spread. When we finally took Ian to the doctor he said it was psoriasis. This was to become another cross for Ian to bear, because it spread to large areas of his body, his scalp and his face.

It is a feature of psoriasis that it comes and goes, and gets worse during periods of stress. When we took Ian to a home so we could have a break for a few days, his psoriasis was always much worse when he came home. So we knew Ian had worried while we were away, even when they told us that he had been good and had enjoyed his stay. This made us feel guilty for leaving him, but you need a break from time to time, to try to behave as a normal family.

Our secretary at work was a Mrs Muriel Boswell, but Brian our accountant always called her Eve, after the singer. As the firm grew and we got more and more large jobs, we had to employ more office staff as well as site workers. Looking back, it is obvious that we were in a building boom. At one time there was a two-year waiting time for delivery on bricks and lots of building materials were difficult to obtain. During the worse time we had Bert Coles in the lorry, spending all day every day going from one builder's merchant to another getting anything that was on offer that day. Some days it might only be two bags of cement or plaster. It became a nightmare trying to keep our sites working.

Over a period of 18 months, the cost of building materials more than doubled and our profits dropped. The problem got so bad that you could only take on a big job if the customer signed an agreement to pay the increase in material and labour costs. They did this by taking the government's weekly price index or listing all the materials and labour you wanted any price increases on. You had to include the current price you had based your tender on. It didn't end there because on the larger sites most builders used sub-contract labour, usually on piece work prices. This meant that you could arrive on site to find a gang of bricklayers or carpenters had vanished, as the site next door had offered two or three pounds more per thousand bricks. The building game was an auction, with prices soaring, as all contracts came with penalty clauses for late completion. All the builders were struggling to complete on time. The effect of this competition was to push up building prices, and the cost of building more than doubled in less than two years.

CHAPTER NINE

Margaret had joined the Women's Institute at Flyford Flavell, and one evening she had gone to a meeting in my car. She was taking back a canning machine, leaving her Mini in case I wanted a car. The local WI had purchased the canning machine to loan out to members, so they could can fruit or veg instead of bottling it. Just after Margaret had gone out, Bill Treadwell came round and told me he had seen a lovely young calf and he would take me to see it if I wanted. He said it was just the other side of Worcester so I agreed. Julie got in the back with Bill, Ian got in the front with me and off we went.

The place was well down in Herefordshire, so it was quite dark when we turned up the narrow lane to the farm. We knocked the farmer up and he took us across the yard to the barn. When he put the light on we saw that he had about twenty calves in the barn. Bill picked out the one he'd told me about and fetched him over, and so I met Fred for the first time. He was a Charolais/ Hereford cross-bred bull calf. I said I would buy him and paid the farmer, promising to come and collect him the next day. He said, 'Take him now or he won't be there tomorrow.' Apparently he had a dealer coming to buy them all the next morning and if he saw Fred he would want him with all the rest. So Bill and Julie got in the back of the Mini, we put a sack over the back end of the calf and laid him on their laps. I settled Ian in the front seat and we set off home. When the calf licked the back of Ian's neck he said, 'Don't like dog'. I don't know if it's any kind of record to take four people and a young cow 30 miles in a Mini, but it felt like it. The inside of the car smelt like a farmyard before we were halfway home and it was days before we got rid of the smell.

That year we had a bonfire party. Bill brought some of his cider so everyone was quite merry. We sat over fifty people that night to eat, even though a lot had to sit on the floor, which gives you some idea of the size of the rooms.

We put the old farmhouse on the market and a blacksmith wanted it as a lot of out-buildings went with it; but he was having trouble getting the mortgage and kept stringing us along. We refused to sell to anyone else as we had promised him he could have it. He let us down when he changed his mind and by the time we got it back on the market, the housing market had collapsed and we ended up dropping the price by £6 000. So we had to take out a mortgage after all. With the interest that had mounted up on the bank loan that we'd got when we were building and trying to sell the house, dropping the price was the last straw. We ended up with a £10 000 mortgage.

Ruth was becoming part of the family as she came every day and spent a lot of time with Magic at the weekends. She was good company for Julie. She also knew where to get the horses shoed and the best places to buy tack and food for them.

One day Julie decided she wanted to buy a donkey with some of the pocket money she had saved, so we found a breeder in Feckenham. When we went to see her she had several young donkeys and she named them all after herbs. The one Julie liked had a long fluffy coat; his name was Parsley and he only cost £45. She just had enough money so she could really feel he was hers. Parsley became part of the family, but he always was a handful, although he was friendly. I think donkeys invented stubbornness: Parsley was big for a donkey and when he got stubborn you couldn't shift him, it would have taken a charge of gunpowder. It became a standing joke in the village and people used to say the children all learned to swear by listening to me cursing Parsley.

We had a felt saddle for him, but no one could ride him. He was like a bucking bronco, he always had them off. The funny thing was that if you put a toddler on his back he was as gentle as a kitten, and when there was a village fete I used to give the young children rides. We always thought that he would tolerate the light weight of young children but not the bigger ones. One day Ruth brought a boy who was older and bigger than Julie, but was blind and had a bad heart. His name was Oliver. Ruth brought him down to hold and touch the animals. When he held Parsley he really loved the feel of him, and asked if he could have a ride. At first I said it was not safe, but Ruth said we could hold Oliver on both sides, so after a lot of pleading I gave in. We tacked Parsley up and Oliver climbed on. My heart was in my mouth for the first few moments, but Parsley was like a lamb and as good as gold. After Oliver had gone the girls tried to ride him, but he was as bad as ever and, try as they might, he was having none of it. The only reason we could think of for Parsley being so gentle with Oliver was that he knew somehow that Oliver had such a severe handicap. Sadly Oliver died a couple of years later.

Early in 1975, someone about three miles away bought a Jenny donkey and Parsley used to shout to her. If you have ever heard a donkey in full cry, you will know what a racket they can make. We recorded him in full flow, and when we played it back to him he went bonkers. I don't know what he was saying, but he certainly didn't like it being said back to him! One day I had him on his halter and told Ian to hold him while I opened a gate that was sticking. It came open with a rush and startled Parsley, who promptly bolted. Poor Ian was still holding and would not let go of the halter, so Parsley dragged him quite a way before I managed to catch them. Ian had a lot of cuts and bruises but luckily nothing serious, and as usual he did not cry.

That Easter Julie invited a friend to stay for a few days. Her name was Amanda but the girls called her Boggy. One day while they were out riding, they were going across the airfield at Throgmorton when an aeroplane started and frightened the ponies. Julie's pony Kate reared up and Boggy had a nasty fall. A passing motorist very kindly stopped and brought them home. Margaret went down to the airfield and asked a passer-by to bring Kate home. She then took Amanda to Pershore Hospital where they said she was too bad for them to deal with and told Margaret to take her to Worcester. I always thought they should have had an ambulance to take her, as the bone was sticking through her skin. She had to suffer all the way to Worcester every time the car hit a bump. Her parents were very angry; I expect we would have felt the same if it had been Julie.

Meanwhile Roy was enjoying himself and making lots of new friends. One night he went to the Church Lench club with Ruth and her friend Anne. They were going with another friend who had a two-seater MG Midget, so it was crowded with four of them in it. We were awakened at 2am by a loud knocking on the door. It was Ruth in a right old panic. She said, 'There's nothing to worry about but we've had an accident and Roy's in hospital.' So was Anne. While Margaret got Ian and Julie up, I had to go and tell the Badhams that their daughter was in hospital. We all went off to Worcester to see what was going on. Luckily the hospital was only keeping them in for observation. They sent Richard home but he was back in hospital a few days later for an operation, as he had broken his cheekbone. So all's well that ends well, but you do tend to worry more when you have a handicapped child and one of the others gets hurt.

That summer we decided to have a holiday, and Julie fancied a riding trip so we booked one in the Mendip Hills in Somerset. Roy didn't want to go so he stayed home and had some of his friends over. Bill Treadwell looked after the animals for us while we were away, and Ian went to Lea Castle for the week. They had opened a short stay home in the Clent Hills and this had the reputation of being the best thing since sliced bread for relief care (I never liked sliced bread either). There were so many things to arrange before we could go away that I began to wonder if it was worthwhile, but finally away we went.

It was a lovely place and the weather was almost too hot. On our first day Margaret and I found out fairly quickly that trotting for several hours on a horse was vastly different from riding a horse across a field at a walk. So Margaret joined some other mothers and stayed on the farm while the kids went riding. My legs had got so bruised that I was not able to ride for a couple of days, but when they went riding across country to Cheddar Gorge I said I would like to go. I was so stiff and sore that, wonderful as it was, it was the last ride I had that holiday.

Back home, we went to collect Ian, but when we arrived at Lea Castle, the person in charge said that we would not be able to take him there again. He said that Ian had behaved very badly and had broken the television set. This, then, was the 'showplace' for relief care. They couldn't even look after our son, who was never destructive at home. It makes you wonder where they got their training in those days. Most places do run things better today, I am glad to say. A few weeks later I decided I would have riding lessons while things were quieter in the winter, so off I went to Moyfield riding stables. I thought if it was good enough for Julie, it was good enough for me.

After the success of Bill's cider at the bonfire party the previous year, we decided we would make our own this year. So we purchased an empty 45-gallon whisky barrel, collected all the windfall apples we could and took them off to Emley Castle to have the juice pressed out. We stood the barrel on a couple of bales of straw, added a little sugar and topped up the barrel every day with water. By Christmas we were able to tap the barrel and enjoy the fruits of our labour, all 45 gallons of it.

Roy was approaching his 17th birthday and I let him drive the car in the field. He had been driving the tractor around the fields for some time, so he had some experience. He took his test after a few lessons and passed first time. To relax I was taking riding lessons and I was also playing darts with Robin for the Boot Inn at Flyford Flavell. Robin was a special constable at Pershore and as they often struggled to put a full team out in the skittle league, Bill and I played for them to make up the numbers when a lot of them were on the late shift. So with an active social life, milking two goats and a cow night and morning, as well as feeding and mucking out the rest of the animals and working nine and ten hours a day, it's no wonder I was as fit as I had ever been.

Early in 1976 I saw a nice pony for sale, a strong ten-year old cob, so I decided to buy him for myself. Windsor Boy was his name. The first day I took him home, I put him in an outside stable with a corrugated iron roof and a five barred gate across the front. The next morning he was out in the field hobbling on three legs, and when I examined him he had a terrible gash on the back of his hock. When the vet came, he said that he was not able to sew it as the skin was too thick where he had cut it. So I had to make a stable in the barn for him, as the vet said we had to keep the cut dry. I had to dress the wound night and morning, dusting it with antibiotic powder. After a few days, Windsor would turn round in his stable when I went in, and hold his leg up for me to attend to. I found out how he had damaged his leg later when I was out riding him. As he jumped, he kicked his hind legs back, which is probably what he had done when he jumped over the five-barred gate to his stable that first night. He must have hit his one back leg on the edge of the corrugated iron roof, cutting it badly.

CHAPTER TEN

One day Margaret and Ian were going out in her car. As she was going down the drive, our gander ran in front of her and she ran it over. When she got out she saw that it was under the Mini, but still alive. She ran to get help and Robin came back with her. He picked up the back end of the car and told her to pull the gander out. When it was free they could not find anything wrong with it, and when they let it go, it ran off. A few days later I noticed the gander had a lump on its back. When I rang the vet he said, 'We don't bother with poultry, just pull its neck.' I didn't want to do that so I thought I would have a look at the damage myself. I set up a trestle table and knocked some nails in to tie the gander to. A full grown gander is a strong bird so I needed to immobilise it if I was going to cut it open. I got Joe, a retired farmer from up the road, to assist and we tied it down. I put Margaret's kitchen gloves on, painted the lump with diluted dettol and cut off the feathers around the lump. I then cut it open with a razor blade and, to my horror, it was full of maggots. The stench was unbelievable. After I cleaned the wound out Joe said it had gone too far. So we took the bird off our operating table and Joe pulled its neck.

After we cleaned up we went round to Robin's to tell him about the operation. As usual there were a few people hanging around talking. That all changed when we appeared in the doorway; as we walked in one end they all disappeared out of the other end of the workshop, complaining bitterly about the smell. I went home, stripped off in the garden, leaving my clothes outside, and went for a shower. Even then the smell hung around me for several days, this amused Ian who delighted in telling anyone he saw: 'Daddy smells'.

Not long after, Bill asked me if he could leave a horse with us for a few days, as he was taking him to market to sell for someone, so I said OK. The morning Bill was due to take the horse, he asked if I would ride him around the field before he loaded him in the box, to quieten him down. Feeling full of myself after taking a few riding lessons, I agreed. We tacked the horse up and off we went. He took off like a rocket, straight down the track towards a five-barred gate. My confidence was leaking like a sieve, and there was no way I was going to jump the gate, so I managed to turn him along the hedge. As he went down the hedgerow like a racehorse, a pigeon flew out of the hedge and startled him. He took a massive leap sideways and reared up, pawing the air like something in a film, and I ended up firmly stuck in the hedge, a hawthorn one at that. I was glad to see the back of that particular horse.

During all this time Ian was having a lot of fits and we had to call the ambulance on a number of occasions when he went into status. It was a great worry, but at least Roy and Julie were old enough to leave at home while we went to the hospital with Ian. The other problem was that Ian would often hurt himself when he fell while going into a fit. The most worrying times were when he hit his head, and he had a lot of nasty bumps because there was no warning when he was about to have a fit.

At other times he was much quieter than he used to be, but still not able to do much for himself. Margaret still had to dress him and take him to the toilet. When Margaret took Julie to Whitford Hall School, Ian always enjoyed travelling in the car and would rock from side to side. This was quite an experience, as the Mini would rock in time with him. There were people who, seeing Ian do this, would mimic him, and it was not always children. We could accept that some children would do it, as they did not know better, but when it was adults making fun of Ian, it really hurt.

Roy was now taking his 'A' levels and Julie was thinking about changing schools, as Whitford Hall only took children up to 12.

For some reason she wanted to go to the Alice Ottley school in Worcester, although all her friends were going to a school in Droitwich. This meant that she had to take an entry exam. She must have done OK, as they accepted her for the September term.

As the summer went on Daisy our Jersey cow calved and everything was fine for a few weeks. We let her feed her calf for about a month and then started to feed him from a bucket of goat's milk. This meant that Margaret and Julie had to get the calf sucking their fingers, then lower their hands into the milk. This was when the calf would suck milk, and after a few days it could feed on its own. We also had to keep the calf with the goats, as he would have helped himself to Daisy's milk if we let him run with her. Sadly, a short while later Daisy's milk yield fell and she became very lethargic. We had the vet in to see her, but after two weeks of treatment we lost her. We were all very upset at losing Daisy, so we decided not to replace for a while, but rely on the goat's milk. The advantage of goat's milk is that you can freeze it. We used to buy one-pint cartons to fill, freeze them and sell them at the gate.

I kept all my tools in the barn and hung the larger ones on nails on the wall. One of these was an adze, which was as sharp as a razor. One day I went to take the scythe down off the wall to cut a patch of nettles down round the back of the barn. As I turned round, the handle of the scythe caught the adze and it fell on my head. I dropped everything and ran to the house, shouting for Margaret with the blood pouring all down my face, neck and over my clothes. She was always much calmer than me in an emergency. She took one look at the state I was in, got a clean tea towel, put it on my head and said to Roy, 'Take your dad to hospital.'

When I got there they said the skin on my head was too thin to stitch, so they put a pressure pad about four inches thick over the wound to stop the bleeding and bandaged round my head and under my chin to hold the pad in place. When they had finished patching me up, I looked like a mummy with four inches of pad on top of my head, and bandage all round my head and face. When we got home I had a rest then went round to see Robin and Bill. They found it very funny, so I got no sympathy there. I was accident prone all my life, so when these things happen it's not totally unexpected. I suppose it stops you getting bored and provides some entertainment for those around you, providing it's not too serious.

The summer of 1976 was one of the hottest on record, and the drought was getting serious. We used to do the hay-making and straw-baling at the weekends to avoid taking time off work. So when it was time to make the hay we would spend 12 or 13 hours a day in the fields. One Sunday, I was watching the news on TV after spending all day throwing bales onto a lorry, and they said that Pershore was the hottest place in Europe that day.

Roy now had his 'A' level results and very good they were. I told him he should take a year out and get a job, as he was only 17. Too many people never leave school; they go straight from school to college, then back to teaching at school. They never know how the rest of us live. So Roy got a job working on the ground with a local grower and driving a small lorry, doing deliveries. I had kept my promise and bought him an old sports car when he was 17. Three of his friends were starting a group and asked Roy to join them. When they had to leave the place they were using to practise, they asked if they could practise in our barn. So I lined the walls of one end of the barn with bales of straw before they started to cut down the noise and avoid upsetting the neighbours. They were a punk group and called themselves Satan's Rats. They started to play at various clubs in and around Evesham. Later they got themselves a manager, who arranged for them to cut a demo disc. This eventually got them a recording contract and they got gigs all over the country.

It was during the summer that we decided it was time Isis, one of our nanny goats, would have to visit the billy goat. The trouble with goats is that it is very difficult to tell when they come into season, at least it was with ours. The billy always knows - well, he would, wouldn't he? So we made some inquires and found someone with a billy goat. They said, 'Bring your goat over and leave her here till the billy serves her'. We borrowed a horse box to take her and we knew we were on the right track when we were within half a mile of the place, as we could smell the billy. They always smell like that so I was glad we did not have our own billy, and I could see why they castrated young male goats.

Later they rang to let us know that Isis was ready to come home, but the horse box was not available. Robin said we could fetch her in the lorry as there was room in the cab. So off we went and on the way back she kept getting her horns stuck in the steering wheel, so I turned her around with her head out of the window. The next thing I heard was Robin swearing as she shit all over his lap. Then, as we came into Upton-on-Severn, we ran into a thick fog. As we were passing the church, a crowd of people were feeling their way along the street and Isis decided to put her head out of the window into someone's face. From the squeal that went up it sounded like a woman. I think she thought the devil was after her. I did check the local papers to see if anyone had suffered a heart attack, but luckily there was no mention of it.

Margaret was now treasurer of the WI so was at least having a night out every week, and getting a break from looking after Ian. Julie was at school in Worcester and caught the school bus at Dormston, which was only three miles up the road. This saved Margaret the long trip to Bromsgrove every day. Ruth was about to start teacher training college and, as she would be living away from home, she decided she would have to sell her horse Magic. This upset her and it took her several weeks to accept it. We missed her while she was away, as she had become part of the family since we had moved to Bishampton.

Ian got a great deal of pleasure from going to the pub and having a drink of beer. We soon learned to buy him his beer in half pints as he would just pour it down his throat. He could down a pint without putting the glass down. It was funny that he took to beer so well, as he only liked very plain food and would not try anything different. He was a chip off the old block there, as I was just the same. I have only ever eaten plain English food, the mere smell of foreign food makes me feel ill.

The only problem with taking Ian out for a meal, which he loved, was that if anyone got served before him, he would want their food. By sod's law Ian was nearly always the last to get his food.

His fits were no better and it seemed such a shame that he should have a fit when he was happy. The trouble was that he could not tell us how he felt after he had a fit, but it appeared to us that he was in pain. We always felt that he must have had severe headaches from the way that he held his head after recovering from a fit. As Ian's vocabulary was very limited, he was unable to tell us if he was in pain, or describe where it was.

We decided we would try to take Ian on holiday with us that year, so we booked a cottage in Cornwall. Roy wanted to stay at home so Margaret, Julie, Ian and I went. Roy looked after the animals with help from Bill Treadwell. We set off on a lovely day in late August and as we went through Devon we started seeing drought notices warning you of the penalties for wasting water.

We got settled in and next day the rains came. For most of the week it rained as if it had never rained before. Still, the accommodation was nice. We spent most of the week travelling around in the car trying to find somewhere to go in the dry. It was not one of our better holidays, proving once again that Ian was happier at home.

CHAPTER ELEVEN

Alcester Builders was growing apace now. We had a surveying department, an estimator and a contracts manager. David was running the office and doing the buying for our sites, while I was concentrating on the maintenance and small works side of the business. I preferred this, as the practical day-to-day work was much more to my liking. I preferred meeting our clients and the closer involvement with the workers to being in the office all day. Most of my men were old hands who had been at the firm all their lives. They were not only employees, they were friends as well (and some still are over 20 years later). On the main contracting side we were pricing much larger jobs and our sites were getting bigger. We were doing a lot of work for the Redditch Development Corporation: houses, schools, old people's bungalows and OAP homes.

One day I had Reg Ainge, one of my team who worked on the small works, come to do some work on the barn. He had his young son Richard with him, who was about six at the time. Richard was playing in the cattle yard when one of the bantam cocks flew at him and racked his face with its spurs. It caused quite a bad cut down his face and just missed his eye, so we decided enough was enough and pulled their necks Jim, one of our foremen, asked if he could have them for the pot. I don't know how he cooked them, but I bet they were very tough. Jim also had the chitlins and the trotters when we killed a pig. I must say, I never fancied them myself.

Late in 1977, Robin and Shirley from next door went to the

70

hunt kennels for the local hunt open day. When they got back Robin came round to see us and said he'd brought us a present. It was a Jack Russell; the hunt were going to put some of them down if they could not find homes for them. We called him Toby and he was a problem from the day we had him. When he first came to us, he had a lot of fleas and in the kennels he'd had to fight for every scrap of food he'd ever had. He was about six months old, so the chances of changing his behaviour were remote, to say the least. All his life he would fight anything that moved, no matter how big, and he lived till he was 17. Rusty, our Staffordshire bull terrier, was a strong dog and over the years we had to mop up a lot of blood. Toby never gave up, he was such a brave little dog. I had trained Rusty well and he would stop fighting when I told him to; otherwise Toby would have had a much shorter life.

It's funny how some years hold better memories than others; 1977 was like that for me. It must have been one of those years when everything goes well, as nothing bad stands out in my mind for that year. We won two large contracts, one for housing at Redditch and one for old people's sheltered housing at Banbury for the Royal British Legion Housing Association.

So as we went into 1978, everything seemed to be going well. Little do we know what the gods have in store for us. Both the contracts were going like clockwork, then suddenly, in the spring of that year, disaster struck. The architect came to do a final inspection at Banbury and it was all passed OK. We had to test the central heating, so we left it on over the weekend. When the men arrived on site Monday morning, the whole place was a shambles. Some of the joints had pulled on the pipework in the roof space, causing water to leak through the ceilings. Most of the ceilings had come down, and the water had ruined the carpets, along with much of the decoration. The architect had nominated the sub-contractors for the plumbing and heating, so this made it their responsibility.

When we contacted the plumbing sub-contractors, they didn't want to know. They said, 'Take us to court.' We then found out that they had no assets. They worked from home and lived in council houses. When we contacted our insurance company, they said that the nominated contractors were responsible. They had no insurance, so as main contractors we were responsible. We then found out that the two men the architect had nominated were so busy they had passed the contract to a mate, who passed it to someone else. Everyone down the line was taking a cut, so the only way the men who did the work could make a living was by cutting corners. At the site meeting with the architects, they said that as they had nominated the plumbers, they would issue the final certificate for full payment if we could rectify the damage in nine weeks. The tenants were due to move in ten weeks later, so we had a rush job on our hands.

We decided the only way we could dry it out and complete the work in time was if I took the small works team down to do it. We were doing 60 to 70 hours a week to get the work done. We had the architect inspect the work half way through the ninth week, and a couple of weeks later they issued the certificate for the full amount due. We still had to pay the cost of doing the repairs, but we were happy that we were going to receive the final payment. When the cheque came the client had stopped seven weeks damages for late completion. This amounted to £42 000, leaving only a little over £7 000 profit. Under contractual law, the client should have paid the amount that the architects had issued the certificate for. The only response we got from the housing association was 'sue us', but things were going too fast for that.

Margaret and I had decided to go away for a few days as it was our 25th wedding anniversary. When we got back I walked into a storm. Our trainee surveyor had overheard the row about money not coming for the Banbury job and when he got to the Redditch job he told everyone about it. Some of the sub-contractors thought we had gone bust, so they started to remove materials off the site. The clerk of works for the Redditch Development Corporation reported what was happening. The result was that they refused to pay the large payment due. After a lot of haggling they did pay nearly half the money they owed us, but the sudden loss of over £100 000 left us with no choice: we asked the band to call the receivers in. This was a mistake as the large firm they sent in were overly expensive and incompetent. They got more than twice what we owed, but took most of it in charges, then lost all the paperwork. This was to go on for nearly six years, during which time the bank said that we owed them £32 000. After a lot of hassle we got them down to £12 000.

The net result of this was that, at 50 years old, I was out of work and the bank had frozen my personal account. So there we were with no money and no prospects. The only chink of light was that I had been looking to start up on my own before all this happened. A firm of building consultants was thinking of taking over Alcester Builders. This meant that I had registered a firm ready to start work. I had some luck and was able to borrow some money from Barclays Bank to start. I asked Paul Quirk and Reg Ainge to work for me, so off we went. I was working on the jobs and doing the pricing and books at night. I got Morag Charman, who used to work at AB, to do my VAT and wages. The only way I could carry on was to raise some money, which meant selling our house and buying something cheaper. I also had a tax demand for £3 500 to cheer me up.

The only bright light was the fact that I never had one word of criticism from Margaret, only help and support, even when we sold the house that she loved. I went to see a thatched cottage in Offenham and fell in love with it. I felt as if I had finally come home. Julie also loved it, but it did not bother Roy one way or another. It took nearly four years before Margaret settled, though Ian fortunately accepted the move as usual with no problems, calling himself 'a cottage boy' once again.

We kept about four and a half acres of the land and the farm buildings. We had to do something about the farm animals; the cats, dogs, Parsley the donkey and Windsor Boy we took with us. We rented some grazing land at Offenham for Parsley and Windsor. As for the goats, poultry and the use of the buildings and land, we let a man from Bishampton have them on loan. One day we had gone to have a look around our land when Toby chased a duck down the ditch and killed it. The funny thing was that he had never touched any of the poultry when we lived there. The next day I went to tell the man we had loaned them to what had happened. Before I could say a word he said, 'We must have had a terrible storm during the night as it drowned one of the ducks.' I did not have the heart to tell him what had really happened.

A few weeks after we moved we went to see if our animals were OK, and got a shock: every one of them had gone. When we went up the village to see the fellow we had lent them to, he was missing too. After much chasing about, we found out that he had sold all our animals and poultry, and gone off to Australia. The thing that worried us most was what had happened to our goats, as we were very fond of them. Things got worse when we found he had sold them to a butcher. When we finally managed to contact the butcher, we had some good news; he had sold them to someone at Bredon. They were in a herd of goats on Bredon Hill and quite content.

I was now using the buildings at Bishampton for storing building materials, so we kept some contact with Robin Shirley and Bill. However, our new life was now in Offenham.

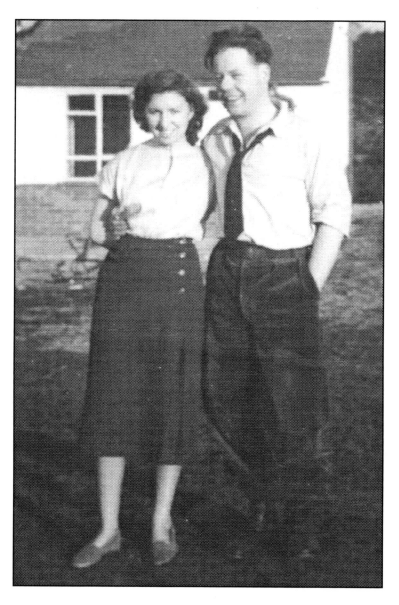

Margaret & Lionel in 1953 just before they married.

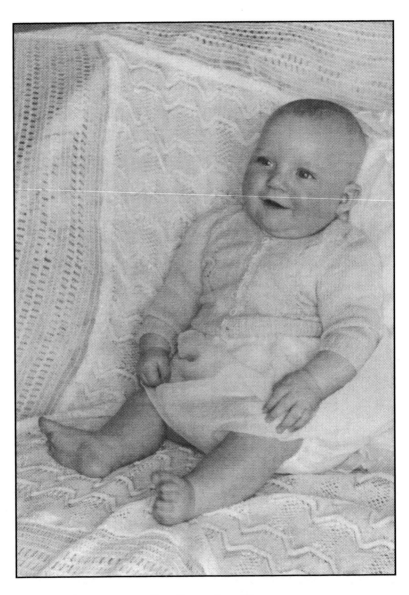

Ian 6 months old.

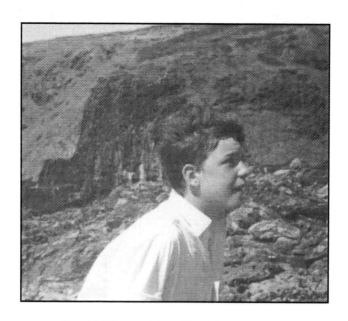

Ian 12 Years old and looking worried
as he often did in his younger years.

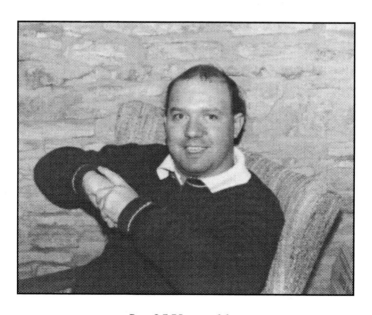

Ian 25 Years old -
On one of his happy days.

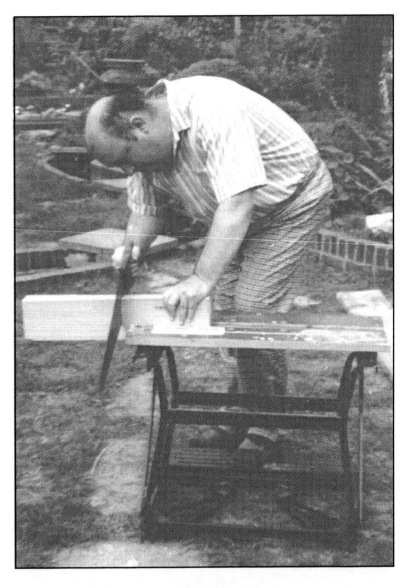

Ian aged 35 -
He enjoyed sawing and knocking nails into wood,
it was one way of working off his frustrations.

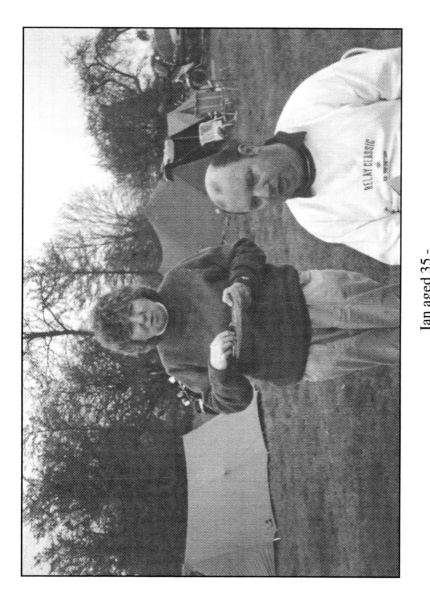

Ian aged 35 -

With Margaret at the Vincent Rally (near Slimbridge Glous.) a few months before we lost Ian.

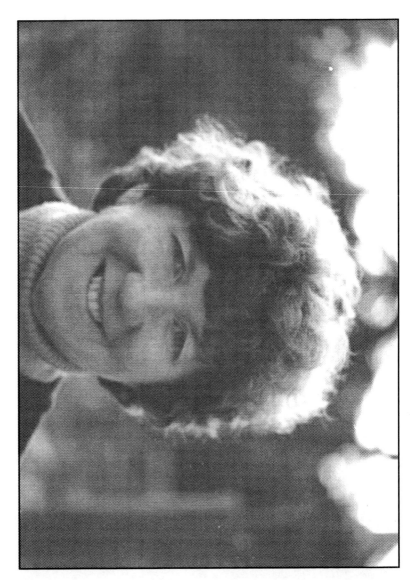

My favourite photograph of my Margaret.

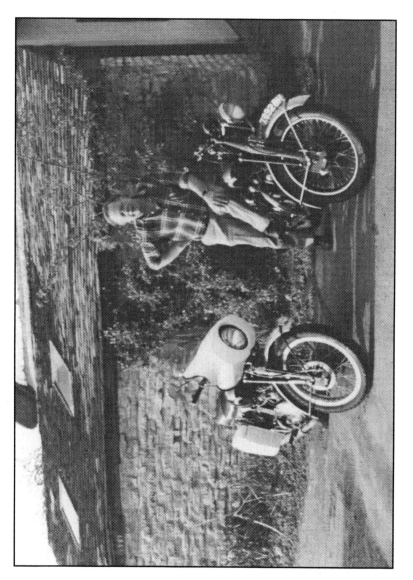

Me with my Vincent HRD Comet & Rapide.

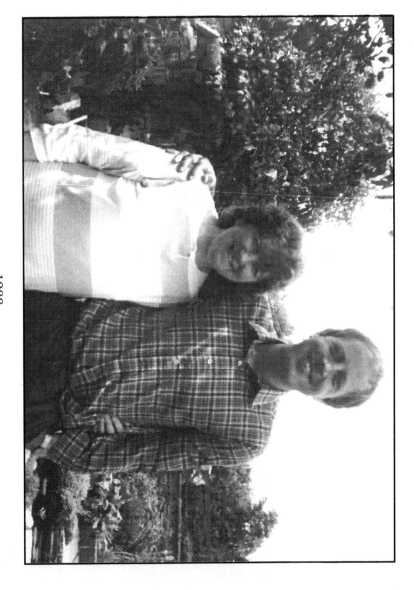

1988
Roy with Margaret.

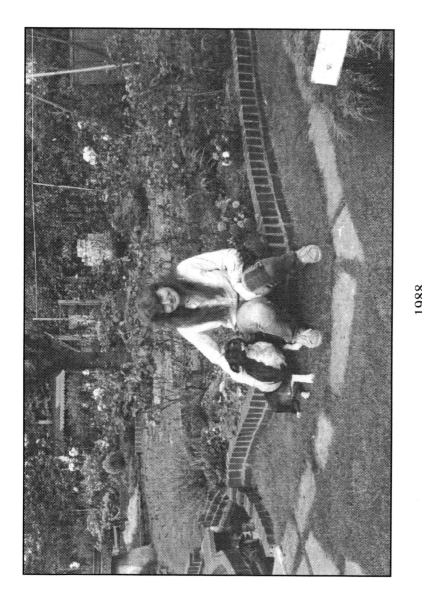

1988

Julie with Pippin, in our garden.

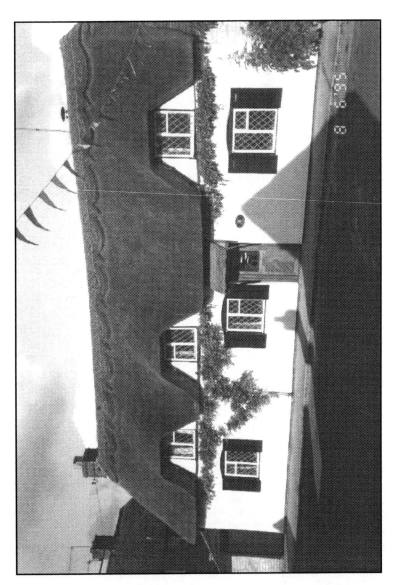

The Old Place -
At the time of the village wake June 1995.

Chapter Twelve

In September 1978 we moved into the Old Place. Things were so different from our previous house with its large rooms and high ceilings. The Old Place had been two cottages for centuries, then after the war someone had converted it into one building. It was a grade two listed building.

The rooms were small (about 14 by 12ft) with low ceilings. That is normal in 500-year old cottages, but it takes some getting used to when you have just moved from a larger house. Ian, however, took to it like a duck to water and soon learned when to duck his head to avoid hitting it on the beams.

I had lots of ideas about how to make the inside more user friendly and open it up. You can alter a listed building inside but not outside without permission. In our restricted financial circumstances, alterations would have to wait till we could afford to do them. I did, though, have to convert part of the conservatory on the back of the cottage into a bedroom for Roy as we needed another one. When we moved in we had an invitation to dinner so we could meet some of our neighbours. Some of the local children came to see if Julie wanted to go to the youth club, which all helped to make us feel welcome, but the big thing was that everyone accepted Ian.

That winter was very cold, but I couldn't understand why it was so cold in the cottage. When I started to look around I found the reason. The dormer windows had been built from bricks laid on edge. Lying in bed one night I noticed that so much of the mortar had fallen out, I could see the cottage over the road through the brickwork. Also, sitting in any of the rooms downstairs, I could feel a draught. So I went round with my bee smoker to find where it was coming from. I found quite a wind coming through the wall in the dining room, a three-foot thick stone wall that had the plaster stripped off to make a nice feature in the room. Fixing it would have meant pointing the wall both sides, and the other side was in next door's cottage, so I decided to insulate the front wall upstairs and down. You need to be in the building business, good at DIY or have a lot of money if you buy a very old cottage. We have been here 20 years now and I am still doing fairly major work. Luckily the men who worked for me before I retired are very good about helping me. The only problem is I have trouble getting them to accept payment.

The good thing about having to do a lot of work in the house was that it amused Ian. He really enjoyed watching me knocking things about, and if things went wrong he would run and tell Margaret, 'Daddy swears.'

We were going into Evesham more now that we were living nearer. The shop assistants and waitresses in the local cafes soon got to know Ian and were very kind to him. There is, however, always the exception. There was one particular man who would follow Margaret and Ian round the town, staring at Ian. This happened on several occasions. As the old saying goes, 'There's nowt so queer as folk'. You just have to not let it get to you.

Not long after we got settled in, we had a visit from the local health visitor, Pearl Barker. She got the social worker Joan Mason to visit us. Joan was a great help, advising us about the benefits that Ian was entitled to and telling us that Margaret could apply for an attendance allowance for looking after Ian. We thought about it and decided that, as we were very hard up at the time, we would go for it. Both women were a great help over the years and became good friends of the family.

That year we were doing some maintenance on the Stratford Canal for the National Trust. They had drained a section of the canal so we could point some brickwork on the locks. There were two main problems: one was the long walk from the road to the lock, the other was the bitter cold wind that seemed to blow straight through the lock. It made for cold and wet working conditions, so it seemed as if you could not get warm before you were back in the wind. Reg Ainge, who had come with me from Alcester Builders, said that his brother-in-law, John Marshall, was looking for a job. I grabbed the chance with both hands as he could help Reg on the canal and I could stay in the warm. John took to the work on the canal like a duck to water. He loved all things to do with the country, and enjoyed working miles from anywhere and anyone.

It was about this time that John Lamburn, our plumber at Alcester Builders, contacted me and asked if I had a job for him. I said yes very quickly, as I knew what a good worker he was. So I now had a workforce of four, which meant I could spend more time finding work and organising things.

We were getting to know our neighbours and most of them were much older than us, though now we are among the oldest in our end of the village. It just shows what 20 years can do!

The first Christmas we were in Offenham, we asked my father to come as usual and spend Christmas with us. Ian and I went to Dayhouse Bank to fetch him on Christmas morning, while Margaret cooked the dinner. He never was very good company - to put it bluntly, he was a bloody misery all his life. When we were young he would keep the front room locked all year, and only open it on Christmas Eve to air the room out for Christmas Day. Then he would spend all day in there on his own, while the rest of the family would sit in the dining room on hard chairs. I don't think I sat in an armchair in our own home till after we got married. But for all that we felt that he shouldn't be on his own over Christmas.

That night we could hear him swearing all night. On Boxing Day morning I asked if he was ill, but he said, 'No, it's this bloody place, it's haunted. I wouldn't spend another night in this house for all the tea in China!' So I took him home that morning and he never spent another night in this cottage. In all the time we have lived here we have never had any such experience. I have always felt that I belong here and that I have finally come home.

As we went into 1979 things started to improve for most of the family, except for poor Ian. If anything, his fits seemed to be getting worse, particularly his night fits. We were still going to Lea Castle for his EEGs (electroencephalograms) and blood tests. The EEGs involved Ian having pads stuck all over his head to pick up the brain waves. He was always very good when they were doing it. (Nowadays, they use a cap with electrodes fixed to it.)

There was a large landing in the cottage that had once been used for a bedroom, with just a curtain to give some privacy. We had Ian sleeping there, so we could be close to him when he had a fit in the night. Luckily Ian had good health generally, but we were still finding it difficult to keep him occupied all the time. Pearl and Joan Mason began trying to get him into the day centre in Evesham that had opened in August 1977. The first response from the day centre and Social Services was that Ian was too difficult for them to handle, and they did not have enough staff. Due to pressure from Pearl and Joan, they finally agreed that the day centre would take Ian for one day a week, starting in September 1979

At first this seemed to be OK, and Margaret enrolled on a typing course at the local tech next door to the day centre. But Ian had problems settling in and they decided that he could only go for half a day a week. The manager was Tony Mann, who had been there for about a year. He said he would try to find a volunteer who would come in one day a week and look after Ian on a one-to-one basis. Ian only went to the centre for a half-day each week for the rest of the year, but at least he did get out for a short time every week.

It was around this time that Roy decided his group was going nowhere, and he would go to university. He got a place at Salford University to start in September, so before we knew where we where, he was off to Manchester. He was lucky to get a place in the halls of residence. The 'year off' that I had suggested he should take had turned into three years. Julie had settled very well at the Alice Ottley school in Worcester and had made a lot of friends.

With the extra workers I now had, I was getting more work in the Warwickshire schools, from Stratford to Henley via Bidford, Alcester and Studley. Most of this work came from Walter Roberts, the county surveyor for that area. We always had a very good working relationship with Walter, as we did with John Goadsby, the building manager for the National Trust in this area.

As we were getting very busy and a lot of our work was small jobs, I decided that it was about time I had someone in the office. I advertised locally and selected Ann Constable from several applicants. She lived in the village so that was a consideration, as she could walk to work. Ann's job was to check the time sheets, work out the costs and submit our invoices, as well as answering the phone. I was spending less time working on site now and more time tendering and buying materials. Although I have always done a lot of hard physical work, I think I must be basically lazy, because I have always been better at telling other people what to do than doing it myself and there is something about watching other people work that appeals to me. Unless, of course, I think they are not doing it correctly, in which case I will say, 'Get out of the bloody way and let me do it.'

Since Ian was down to half a day a week at the day centre, Joan Mason suggested that we took him to a small unit in Bath Road, Worcester to see if they could take him for one day a week. Bath Road was a residential home with a workroom in the basement to occupy some of the residents. There were about nine or ten residents with only two staff and some volunteers to help. When we first went there, they were knitting and pegging rugs, so my first reaction was: 'This won't be suitable for Ian.' Wendy, who was in charge, soon put me right and explained that they would be able to occupy Ian. He could draw and use Plasticine, so we said we would try it.

They were wonderful with Ian and we were never able to thank them enough for all their efforts with him. The only problem was that access to the building was down a flight of steep steps on the outside; but at least they had constructed a veranda over them to give weather protection. It always worried me having to take Ian down those steep stairs, because he was such a big fellow. He weighed over 14 stone and if he slipped he could have really hurt himself.

It was early in 1980 that Tony Mann told us he had found a volunteer to look after Ian for one day a week. Her name was Ann Causier. We arranged to take Ian for a full day, wondering how long Ann would cope with him as she had not worked with handicapped people before. As it turned out, she had a natural ability for working with people like Ian, and is now, nearly 20 years later, in charge of the special care unit at the day centre. This did not exist then, of course, as the local authority insisted there was no call for one. People like Ian did not exist, as far as the top brass in the Social Services were concerned. Or, worse still, he was acknowledged but ignored. All this meant that we were taking Ian to Worcester and collecting him once a week, as well as taking him to the day centre in Evesham. We also had to take Julie to the station in Evesham every morning to catch the train at 8am, and collect her in the afternoon. Most of the transporting still fell on Margaret's shoulders, as I had to stay by the phone to deal with any calls. We were still using a battered old Mini and two clapped-out vans to run the business, so Margaret and I had to share the Mini, which sometimes caused problems.

I decided to buy a new pickup, but then found problems in getting HP as I only had one year's financial accounts. I spent a couple of hours on the phone and found a large company who would fund the purchase at a very good rate of interest. This taught me a very valuable lesson, and after that I always spent time on the phone when buying materials for our contract work. By doing this, I reckon I saved a lot of money over the years, and when the business got bigger I employed someone to spend most of their time chasing prices. We were doing small contract work through the summer, as well as the maintenance work. The chaps I had working for me were always polite and did a good job, which meant that our firm, Leon Building Services, was much in demand.

John Marshall, who was now doing our brickwork, was a taxidermist in his spare time. He had started as a boy and was now very good. When he was working on the canal I would sometimes take his wages to his house to save going up the canal. One day I went to his house to leave his wages and his wife Frances asked me in for a cup of tea. When I went in, I had the shock of my life: on either side of the fire place there was a stuffed leopard! When I commented on them, Frances took me to see the deep freeze. When she opened it I had another shock, as it was full of penguins waiting to be stuffed. John did them all on the kitchen table. A few years later he left Leon's to take up taxidermy full time. The local council were very good and rehoused him in a larger council house with a big garden so he could build a workshop. John has made a success of his venture and is still doing it today, although he now only does fish.

During the winter Julie had taken up rowing, and was asked to row in the ladies' four. It wasn't until Julie started rowing that I realised how strenuous a sport it is and the amount of training involved. They had a very good crew and started to make an impression in the heats of the river races. They had an even better summer, winning a lot of races. We still have a box full of trophies at home. At first the son of one of the rowers was coxing for them and then Julie asked a school friend, Carol, to do it, as she was quite petite. She was very successful at it and coxed for the Cambridge crew some years later, when they won the boat race for the first time in years. I still remember watching it on TV when the umpire was shouting at Cambridge to move over.

Julie was 17 now and wanted her driving licence, so after a few lessons I started to go to more of the races with her and let her drive. As a lot of the races were all over the country, she got plenty of practice. One day she asked to borrow the car, a new Ford Capri that we'd had for only a month. She said her boyfriend Andy had got a full licence and would go with her. So early Sunday morning they went to Derby for a race. That evening she came through the door and said, 'Dad, I've got something to tell you. I've had an accident and smashed the car.' I said, 'Are you both OK then?' She went off the deep end at me, saying, 'I've been worried all day that you were going to go mad and all you can say is, are you OK!' It turned out that when they were going through our village, a car came out of a small road and smashed into the side of our car. It had happened only two hundred yards up the road from our house but they'd carried on to Derby anyway. So if Julie worried all day it was no more than she deserved.

CHAPTER THIRTEEN

For the New Year of 1981, we told our neighbours that we were having an open house to let the new year in. Most of the people who came were the older ones who were on their own; most of then have passed on now. Still we had a very nice time and did the same for the next few years.

Ann Constable now came for four half days a week and stayed with us till I retired at the end of 1994. I now had Reg Ainge and John Lamburn mainly doing maintenance work for the National Trust and Warwickshire County Council. Paul Quirke and John Marshall were doing the small contract work, and when we did a small extension and needed the rooms plastering, I contacted Geoff Hands who had worked for me at Alcester Builders. After a few jobs Geoff came to work for me full-time and stayed till I retired. So with the business now doing well we were getting back on our feet.

Roy had settled in Manchester and met Paula at the university, where he got very involved in the anti-nuclear campaign. One day they told us they were getting married. The wedding was to be in Paula's home town of Glasgow. The day before the wedding Margaret, Julie, Ian and I set off for Glasgow. We got bed and breakfast just outside the city and next morning set out to find the registry office for the wedding. I should have got a taxi, as we wasted a lot of time chasing round trying to find it. We finally found it just in time. Roy was outside looking for us and getting worried in case we didn't arrive in time. He was there with Paula's sister, Mom and Gran. We were meeting Paula's family and friends for the first time. The ceremony went off well and after taking some photos we went to Paula's mum's for a snack then we set off for home. Ian was as good as gold all the time, but then he always loved Roy and enjoyed travelling, so it was like a holiday for him.

When we moved to Offenham we had rented some land to graze Parsley and Windsor Boy, who Julie was now riding. As she was now in the sixth form and studying for her 'A' levels as well as meeting her rowing commitments, we decided to take Parsley and Windsor back to Bishampton. What with the travelling to look after them, Windsor's gift for jumping fences and the complaints we were getting from the neighbours, we reluctantly decided that we would have to sell him and Parsley. This was quite a wrench as they were the last link with all our animals, except the dogs Rusty and Toby.

At this time I was using the pickup to run round the jobs and take the materials. Paul had a clapped-out old van and took John with him. Geoff and Reg used their own cars, while John had the old Mini van. We were desperate for more vehicles and I ended up buying two second-hand Astra vans which were only a few months old. This meant that Margaret had our car to take Ian out and drive him to the day centre and Worcester.

With Ian going to the day centre one day a week, we started to get involved and went to the open days and events that the staff organised. We soon noticed the other parents' lack of interest in the running of the centre. This meant that the staff were always struggling to get parents on the support group committee, so I soon got talked into joining them. We were very lucky to have Ken Fletcher as our chairman, and he was prepared to put a lot of his spare time into doing the job.

The committee decided to raise some money to open a special care unit at the day centre. The total lack of support for the project from Social Services left us with no option but to try and raise the funds ourselves. We tried organising some events but the money we collected was just a drop in the ocean. We then started writing to various local organisations to try and get support, and some gave us a great deal. For example, the Round of Gras in Badsey raised nearly £2000. On the other hand, the British Legion in our village informed us that they did not support charities, although I was at that time a member - not for long after that! (Other branches of the Legion did support the cause, however.) We started looking into the possibility of raising enough money in the September of 1981, though we were well into 1982 before we started our fund raising.

In January Paula had our first grandchild, a little girl called Jenny. So Roy was now a father and about to take his finals at university. He got an honours degree. As he and Paula had decided to stay in Manchester, he had to try and find a job to support his family - not as easy as it sounds, even if you had a good degree, as jobs were very scarce in the north around that time. He ended up working in a factory making asbestos brake linings, which worried Margaret and me as the asbestos scare was just starting. But the young don't see the dangers that we oldies see.

In the March of 1982 Julie was 18 and had a party at a pub in Pershore. It was a toga party and all her friends arrived on a cold night, wrapped in sheets and little else. Ian was staying at a place in Dudley for the weekend, and Margaret and I booked in at a hotel in Evesham overnight so we would be out of the way when a crowd came home from the party.

The year wore on and Julie took her 'A' levels. She was offered several places to take her degree, but wanted to go to Bristol where her boyfriend Andy was going. It was all a last minute rush and they kept dashing about looking for accommodation, but all the halls of residence places had gone. She finally settled into her four-year course in Applied Biological Sciences.

By this time our fundraising was underway and Tony Mann, the day centre manager, told us he was going on a two-year course. A John Curren would be taking over as manager in his absence. John was a great help with our fundraising and attended all our meetings, which were now held nearly every week.

That summer I had purchased a Vincent Comet motorcycle made in 1951 and decided to ride from John o'Groats to Land's

End as a sponsored event. With the help of the local paper and pressure on all our friends, I got some sponsors and raised over £700 towards our funds for the special care unit. People say it's not far, but on your own in all sorts of weather, it seems twice as far as it is. I remember sitting under the railway bridge at Gloucester for two hours while the heavens opened. I had to get all my clothes dried at my Cornish bed and breakfast, right down to my pants and vest. Oh, the pleasures of the open road!

Margaret had been having a few medical problems lately and the doctor sent her to see a specialist. We were in BUPA at the time so we were able to see him quickly. He told us Margaret would have to have a hysterectomy, and arranged for her to have it done at the Nuffield Hospital in Cheltenham. We didn't have long to make our arrangements. The first priority was to find somewhere for Ian to stay for a couple of weeks. The Social Services told us about a home just outside Worcester that might accept Ian for a short time. We went to look around and let them meet Ian.

When the manager showed us around the home, the first thing we noticed were that they had given all the residents some jobs to do. He would say, 'Tommy, go and dig up some potatoes for dinner' and then 'Betty, will you change the sheets on the beds'. I told him Ian was not like the other residents and wouldn't be able to help like them. He said, 'We are professionals and know to handle all types of handicapped people.' Srangely, Ian was unusually well behaved that day.

The next week we took Ian to the home on Tuesday morning and settled him in, then I took Margaret to the hospital and stayed while she got settled. They were doing the operation the next day, and she looked very poorly when I saw her afterwards.

On Thursday morning, just after I opened the office, I had a phone call from the manager of the home where we had left Ian. He said, 'You'll have to come straight over and collect Ian. He is uncontrollable, he ripped his sheets in the night and we can't put up with that.' I said I wouldn't be able to collect him till late afternoon as I had some appointments, but would come about 5pm. The only thing I could think of was that he had gone into a very bad fit in the night. If that was the case, they should have had someone on duty to attend to him, or perhaps they were using old and rotten sheets. When I got home at lunchtime, the staff were sitting outside our house with Ian in their car. The first thing they said to me when they got out of the car was, 'We are not prepared to wait for you to collect him.' So much for the so-called professionals. They should have tried looking after him when he was younger, then they would have known what uncontrollable meant.

That evening, when I went to visit Margaret she had quite a shock when she saw Ian, and couldn't believe it when I told her what had happened. Julie arrived a short time later to see her mum, as it was not far from Bristol by car. After we had been there about an hour, a nurse came to change the bag that was draining the operation wound. When she replaced it, I heard something and turned round to see Julie sliding down the radiator; she had fainted!

A few days later when Margaret was starting to get out of bed, she had a spell of discomfort and couldn't settle at night. For a couple of nights the staff found her wandering round the hospital corridors, not knowing where she was: some sort of sleep-walking, I suppose. When she came out of hospital the doctor told her not to do any hoovering or cleaning for some months, so we had to get someone to help in the house. When I asked around, Ann who worked for me in the office said she knew someone suitable. Pat Hill lived at the other end of the village, and she had two girls Sam and Steph, who were eight and six at the time. Pat was bringing the girls up on her own after separating from her husband, and she needed the money. She came in two mornings a week to do the housework until Margaret was able to do more. Then I got Pat to clean the office as well as helping Margaret, as there was no way we were going to lose her. She was such a lovely person and soon became one of the family, like another daughter. All these years later, she still comes to dinner every week to cheer us up.

Christmas '82 was soon on us and, as Margaret was feeling a lot more mobile, we were able to go up to Roy's and see how our lovely new granddaughter was getting on. Julie was, of course, home for the holidays. Ian had a lovely time, as he was well and not having as many fits. He never quite understood the concept of Christmas presents, so we had to give him his gifts one at a time over several days. I suppose we could have just bought him a few things, but we tended to go over the top, like most parents, and buy him loads.

Ian was often unwell at Christmas. With someone like our Ian, you never knew if it was the excitement of seeing all the family and the build-up to Christmas that brought on the fits, or if it was just one of his normal periods of being unwell. It's such a shame, as it means you can't plan ahead. Take the year we booked a Christmas day dinner at a pub. Halfway through the starter Ian started to have a fit, and a short while later, as they were bringing the main course, he had another. He was so poorly that we had to help him to the car, take him home and lay him down. Although our rooms are on the small side, we have always had three-seater settees so that Ian could lie down and be with us.

He was getting to be a big man now, so he took some handling when he was poorly. One of his few pleasures in life was food. He really enjoyed it, so we indulged him. I suppose we made things worse in a way, but we have no regrets, at least he had some pleasure in his short life. I hate to think how we would have felt if we had kept him on a diet all those years.

CHAPTER FOURTEEN

A s we went into 1983, our fundraising was coming on well and we made our first approaches to Social Services, whose first response was that there were not enough people in the day centre catchment area to warrant the expense. So we started our own survey to find out how many had been excluded from the centre on the same grounds as Ian, that is, because they were too difficult. In the centre's catchment area we found 32 families who were getting no day care for their dependents. We spent all of that year and a lot of 1984 without getting any positive response. Our chairman Ken was a tower of strength during our battles with Social Services. He worked on the principle that dripping water could wear away stone. Had it been me dealing with them, I would have used dynamite and probably got nowhere.

As the business was still doing well and I had Paul as foreman, we decided to take a holiday that spring. After a lot of sorting around we decided on a week in Scotland with Shearing Coaches. We arranged for Ian to stay at Himley House in Dudley, a home for about ten residents run by a family who lived on site. They were quite good with Ian so we went off that Spring feeling happy that he was being well cared for.

The coach collected people as it went north. A couple from Bradford, Colin and Doreen Scarbrough, got on and sat in front of us, and during the trip we got to know them well. We were to enjoy several holidays with them over the next few years. We stayed part of the time at the Dunblane Hydro, a huge Victorian hotel. We were not used to the sort of luxury they offered. That first holiday in Scotland I fell in love with the landscape and people, and this was the first of many visits we made to the Highlands and Islands.

When we got home and collected Ian, he was so happy to be home that we felt guilty about going on holiday and leaving him. So a few weeks later we tried taking him away for the weekend. We did take him to the seaside from time to time for the day, but had not stayed away overnight with him for quite a long time. We went to Minehead and got bed and breakfast, but although he was quite happy during the day he was not too happy about staying overnight. As usual he was only really happy when we got home and he walked into the cottage.

Of course it was always difficult with him having fits when we were out. If we were local we could get him back in the car and home, but if we were a long way away that was a problem. Most days I tried to get home for dinner so I could take Ian and the dogs for a walk up the hills. When Margaret came with me it was OK, but if I took them on my own it could be awkward, as Ian did not walk very well. If he had a fit while I was out on the hills with him, I was up shit creek without a paddle. I waited till he recovered, then I had to assist him back to the car over some very rough ground. Margaret was always very worried if we got home late, and after that episode she always asked where we were going so she could come to help if we were a long time.

By this time I had a Polish carpenter working for me. His name was Alex Wolski and he had about 16 acres of land at the top of the hill, which had better access to the road. So when I had Ian with me and we took the dogs, we went there for our walk.

One day I had taken Ian, Rusty and Toby out for a walk. While we were out we met someone with a large dog and, as usual, Toby was in like a dose of salts and a fight was soon in progress. I was struggling to hold Rusty, who wanted to go and help Toby. The big dog picked Toby up by the scruff of the neck and shook him like a rat. He then ran into the woods with him. So I took Ian and Rusty home and told Margaret to get a bucket and shovel so we could go and find what was left of Toby and scrape him up. We were just about to go when in walked Toby as if nothing had happened, with hardly a mark on him. Alex had found him and brought him home.

Of all the dogs we ever had, most of which were Staffordshire bull terriers, Toby was the only aggressive one. He was generally good with people and children, but seemed to take a dislike to certain adults, such as Paul Quirke. If Paul came into the garden, Toby would sneak up behind him and bounce up and down, biting Paul's backside; but like most builders, a few rips in his jeans didn't make much difference to Paul. If we were out walking with him and any bulls or horses came up to us (as they do), Toby would round them up and chase them away. In some ways he was a nightmare, but he was so loyal and had so much character that he more than made up for his misdemeanours.

By now Julie had got rid of her car, so I started looking for a motorbike for her, and saw an old 250 BSA Starfire advertised in Evesham. When I tried out the bike, I found that it went like shit off a shovel, as the saying goes, which surprised me. The man who was selling it, Norman Best, was into old bikes. So we got to know him quite well, and became good friends over the years. Julie took the bike to Bristol and joined the local BSA club, and when the Classic Bike show was on in Bristol that year, Julie's bike was in the show. I went for the day. While I was looking round the exhibits I saw the Vincent Stand and went over to talk to them. There I met Jack Barker from Dursley for the first time, who was to become a very good friend and a great help rebuilding several of my motorbikes over the years.

Our local Friends of the Earth group collected waste paper for recycling every month in the Oat Street car park in Evesham. As we were already in Greenpeace, we got involved by transporting the paper to a house in Broadway Road for storage. Ian would come with me as he really enjoyed sitting in the pickup while I drove around. He also enjoyed the company and would rock back and forth, making the pickup rock in time with him.

Since Ian was at home so much, it was always difficult to keep him occupied. He was not capable of doing much and would soon

91

get bored when Margaret got him to draw or do any other activity. He could not concentrate for very long. Margaret would take him to the shops two or three times a week to buy him a little matchbox car and take him for a cup of tea and a doughnut. He always insisted that the 'lady' had given him the car. All he would do with them was hold them, and at one time he had to have cars with opening doors so he could put his thumb and finger in them. As a result of, we still have boxes of cars; we usually give a few away when there is a local fund-raising or Mencap event.

Roy, Paula and our lovely little granddaughter Jenny had settled in North Manchester, and Roy had applied to join the fire service, as there were no jobs about at that time in the north. It was a good job that he had kept himself fit, as the training was gruelling and a lot of trainees dropped out. What surprised me was the amount of building knowledge they had to learn. Thinking about it, though, it made sense as they didn't want burning buildings falling on top of them in an emergency. We would go up to Manchester to see Roy and family fairly regularly, and Ian always got very excited about going to see them. We have always taken a lot of pleasure from the way that Jenny, then Emma when she came along, treated Ian as if there was nothing different about him. They just accepted him.

The year was rolling by and Ian was still only getting two days a week day care. We were despairing of getting any help with him. He needed to get away from the house to try and improve his general living skills, such as using a knife and fork, dressing and undressing and going to the toilet on his own. Someone with Ian's degree of disability requires specialist training just to acquire basic skills.

It was just before Christmas that Joan Mason told us of a scheme to give carers the odd night out. They named it Crossroads, after the TV series of the same name. The actors and workers on the programme had raised the money to get it off the ground. They'd had the idea of employing people to come into your home and offer a little help, like helping to give a bath to handicapped people or looking after them while their carers had an evening out. We said great, we would like to try it.

So early in 1984 the organiser from Worcester came to see us, then she brought a lady named Margaret from Harvington to see us and meet Ian. She arranged to come two or three times initially to get to know Ian. At first she was just going to stay two hours to make sure he was OK. The night came, we got dressed up and when Margaret arrived we set off with great hopes. The only problem was that we had not decided what to do; it had been so long since we'd had a night out that we didn't know where to go. So we drove to the top of the Fish and Anchor Hill just outside our village and parked the car. We sat there for nearly two hours, spending most of the time worrying if Margaret was coping OK with Ian. Then we went home and found him enjoying himself, so we'd worried for nothing. The next time Margaret came, we made sure we knew where we were going in advance. She was a lovely lady and Ian grew really fond of her. Little did we know that she would develop cancer about 12 months later. She lost the battle after a few months and died, so we lost a new but cherished friend.

We had been putting pressure on Social Services throughout 1983 by getting articles published in the local press, as well as writing letters to our MP, Social Services and the regional health services. Soon we had raised enough money to build a special care unit and we asked the Social Services to employ one full-time and two part-time instructors. Finally, in February 1984, they appointed Shirley Howsen in charge of special care, with Heather and Rachel as part-time assistants. They had to move around the day centre to any room that was not in use, carrying all their equipment on a trolley, which was not a very satisfactory arrangement. They could only have Ian three days a week, but they did arrange to collect him from home on the mini-bus. The bus had an escort as well as a driver, so we were quite happy for him to travel that way. We arranged for him to go to the Bath Road centre the other two days, where we still had to take and collect him.

We had a letter from Shirley after Ian's first day, telling us what he had done. He had painted in the morning, had his dinner, then spent some time doing a simple jigsaw, though he could only manage two pieces without assistance. We got another letter the next week, then Shirley started a diary which they filled in every week for Ian to bring home on Fridays. Margaret would fill in the details of his weekend; the first one was 2 March, 1984. This meant that we could talk to him about what he had done at the centre and they could talk to him about what he'd done at home. Reading those diaries now brings a lot of things back. I remember two little girls, Anna and Melanie, who used to come to our cottage to play with the dogs and take them for walks. Like most children the girls were very tolerant of Ian and did not seem to find him strange. They would draw for him, or do his simple jigsaws for him. Ian would get very excited if anyone did things for him and say: 'Who's mummy or daddy now?'

Early in 1984 Jack Barker asked me to go to the Vincent winter rally in Holland with him. As it was winter we went in my car and I had my first experience of travelling on the European mainland. To put it mildly, I was hooked. Then that Easter I booked a long weekend in Paris for Margaret and me with a local coach firm. We had a lovely time and after years of saying that I never wanted to go abroad, I was keen to see more.

About three years earlier I had gone to the doctor with severe chest pains. His response was that it might be indigestion, so I should take some anti-acid and if it did not work, start taking angina medication. When I got home and thought about it, I said to Margaret, 'I am not standing for this', so I booked a medical at the BUPA centre in London. I was so impressed, it was like another world. They treated me like a human being for a change and the doctors did not act like they were some superior beings. Ever since then, I had been trying to get Margaret to go, but no way would she agree. So when we were on our way back from Paris and Margaret was saying what a lovely time we'd had, I said, 'We're having a day in London the day after tomorrow.' 'That would be great,' she said, 'what is it in aid of?' So I told her I had booked a medical for both of us.

On Thursday we went to London and as the ladies' medical centre was in a different part of the city, I took Margaret first then

94

went to have mine. As women's plumbing is different from men's, the ladies' medical takes a little longer than the men's. I had expected her to be waiting when I got back as I had travelled across London and back. When I got there they told me she would be a little longer, as they had to do some more tests. When Margaret finally arrived in the waiting room, she looked shocked and told me they had found a lump in her breast. We were a bit down on the way home, and we were on tenterhooks waiting for the letter to say when she was to go to hospital.

After two weeks we had a letter asking her to go to the Nuffield Hospital in Cheltenham. The surgeon who did the operation removed the lump and sent it for biopsy. When we went to see him for the results he informed us that it was malignant, and Margaret would have to go for chemotherapy. She had to go to Cheltenham General Hospital for five treatments a week for six weeks, which made her feel very low, but she put a brave face on. I could see in her face and eyes that she was suffering, but would she admit it? Not on your Nelly. She had a check-up every month for six months, then every three months for a further year, followed by every six months for about the next three years. The funny thing was that after the operation, I knew without doubt that she would make a full recovery, which, thank God, she did. How she went through it all and still coped with Ian, I will never know.

CHAPTER FIFTEEN

Julie had now done two years at college and had started her one-year practical work. They found her a placement at the MAFF in Guildford. I think they had about three students there and they were always up to some trick or other. She made some good friends and still meets some of them now. Once again Pat was proving a Godsend, helping out while Margaret was going to the hospital every day. She came every week to clean the office and help with our housework. She was now stopping to dinner every week when she came to do the work; she was always so cheerful and bright and Ian loved her company. The couple in the cottage opposite left to go and live in Wales and Annie and Alan Gibson moved in. Annie was soon coming over on a regular basis, mainly when Pat was here and between them they made the cottage come alive. This was good for Ian as he loved the talk and laughter and was more animated while they were here, rocking from side to side and singing, putting his own words to the tunes unless he'd had one of his fits, of course, and then he was very lethargic.

At the day centre the more capable clients used to do pottery and woodwork. One day, watching them sawing wood for bird houses, I thought: Ian could do that. So that weekend I got some 4 by 2 and showed him how to saw it. I was surprised how quickly he got the idea; the only problem was that when he had sawn one piece he had no interest in doing another. He would say, 'Ian's sawn the wood' if I tried to get him to cut another piece. He was very proud of having cut the wood and would run to his mom to show her what he had done. At least it was another way of occupying him. The next thing I tried was knocking some four-inch nails about half an inch into a log and getting Ian to knock them right in. I know a lot of people who can't knock a nail in without bending it but Ian could, and he really enjoyed doing it. He probably got rid of a lot of his frustrations that way. With Ian going to Evesham and Worcester five days a week, we began to realise that you can have a handicapped son and still have some life of your own.

As I get further into Ian's diary, I recall more of his funny little ways, and other things of interest. For example, Pearl used to go to the day centre to take a sample of Ian's blood on a regular basis, to monitor how effective his drugs were. He was on so many tablets it was a wonder he didn't rattle every time he moved, and they were still not controlling his fits. If we had been working in a residential home looking after Ian, we would have to have had training to administer his drugs, especially the valium pessaries that we had to use when he went into status. I feel someone should have given us first aid training, not just told us to put him in the recovery position without even showing us what it was. Luckily I took a first aid course and I had been a weight-lifter when I was younger, so I knew how to move him when he required help as he recovered.

We bought a motor caravan and our first trip was to Weston for the day. When we parked on the front, the parking attendant impressed me very much. When I went to pay he noticed Ian and said that parking was free for the handicapped. I explained we didn't have a handicapped pass but he just put a note on the windscreen and refused payment. It's these little things that help so much and make you realise that people do care.

We were looking after Jenny that week so she was enjoying playing on the sand and in the sea. Ian was having more fun watching her play and when she squealed he thought it marvellous and got very excited. He got the most pleasure from having fish and chips for lunch and going to a pub for a pint of beer. As there was a bed in the back of the caravan, he was able to lie down on the journey home. We did try staying overnight once in the Forest of Dean, but it was not a success as Ian wanted to be at home in his own bed. Then to make matters worse it rained overnight and we could not get off the site, so we had to wait for a tractor to tow us off. The main advantage in having it was that when Ian had a fit, we could lay him down and if he was still poorly after a while we could drive home with Margaret in the back looking after him. The motor caravan was a fairly old one but it served its purpose, and allowed us to take Ian out more and further.

Ian was 27 years old now and for the first time in his life he was being taught basic living skills, as his first review shows. This review says that he attended the centre on Monday, Thursday and Friday, that we were taking him and he came home on the bus. It mentions that the other clients tended to make a great fuss of Ian and wanted to do everything for him. This caused a problem as the whole idea was for Ian to learn to do things for himself. We could appreciate how frustrating it was, watching him struggle to do even the simplest tasks. It was much easier to do them for him, but that was not the object of the exercise. I have included extracts from this review just to show his ability.

Self care: Ian can feed himself with a fork but is unable to use a knife. He requires assistance to collect his cutlery and lunch tray.

Toileting: Ian asks when he wants to use the toilet, but needs help to undo and fasten his trousers and requires verbal prompts.

Washing: Ian is reluctant to wash his hands and needs physical guidance, but can dry them.

Dressing/undressing: Ian requires physical assistance with this so it presents an opportunity to work in this area.

Social skills: When you give Ian the choice of two activities, it is difficult to get him to answer. He may just point at something. He also finds it difficult to find his way round the centre, but he knows where the dining room is. (Trust Ian to find food!) At first he would hold his hand out for you to lead him everywhere, but now no longer does this. Ian does not interact with other people at the centre and you have to encourage him to respond to a greeting. On an individual basis Ian responds and can be quite amusing. His family are very important to him and he will always talk about them.

Language: Ian's language is good, he can understand simple instructions. Generally he does not name objects when asked but will sometimes repeat words. He can ask if he wants something, If he wants the toilet, or his car or book.

Cognitive skills: Ian can draw or paint on his own, and can cut out a picture very roughly. He can do inset puzzles or thread beads with assistance. He can match some objects but not colours.

Practical skills: Ian can take his coat off and hang it up if prompted. We are encouraging him to collect his own drink at break times and his own lunch. The other clients used to do this for him and it has taken some time to change this. He will also fetch and carry things if requested.

Motor skills and activities: Ian walks well, he can manage stairs without difficulty. He likes to go out enjoys going to a cafe for a drink.

Targets: We are aiming to enable Ian to become more independent. This will include him collecting his own drink and returning his own cup, setting his own place at the table and collecting his own lunch, collecting his own coat at the end of the day and walking to the bus unescorted. In the self care areas we will concentrate on washing hands, dressing and undressing.

Ian's toe and fingernails were getting very thick due to his psoriasis, which also covered other parts of his body, particularly his scalp, under his arms and between his legs. This meant rubbing ointment into the affected areas before shampooing his hair and bathing him. He loved having a bath or shower but was not too fond of having his hair washed. All his clothes had to be of a non-irritant material, cotton mostly, at least next to the skin. We also had to have his shoes made to measure as he had wide feet and because of the state of his toenails. Ian had his big toenail removed as it was ingrowing, due, we felt, to the difficulty of obtaining wide-fitting shoes for him. Of course Ian could not tell us when his shoes hurt him, and we would not know until we saw blisters on his feet. Having shoes made is a costly business, but it was worth it, knowing that Ian was not in pain.

Ian also suffered from constipation and Margaret found that he was better if he only had wholemeal bread. One of the problems was that he was very reluctant to eat vegetables and the only way Margaret could get any down him was to make vegetable soup. Generally it seemed to work, which was a good job as he also had piles that would bleed from time to time.

I hope I am not painting too bleak a picture of life with Ian, because we did have a lot of fun with him, especially when he was in one of his good moods. He could have us laughing our socks off with some of his comments. If there was anyone about who didn't know Ian, they would be quite bemused at the antics we got up to. Whenever Roy and family or Julie came home, Ian would get so excited that he would start to have fits, which was such a shame as he could take a couple of days to recover.

At this stage of his life I would say that he was happy and in reasonable health for 75% or 80% of the time. A lot of this was due to the time that Margaret spent occupying him. It was not as if he could sit and watch television, so he would listen to his records if he was in the right mood, rocking from side to side.

CHAPTER SIXTEEN

At the day centre we finally got to see the drawings for the new special care unit that they were going to build alongside the existing day centre. So 1985 looked like it was going to be a good year. At home the business was still going well, and I had taken on a part-time office worker, Angie Haughty, who also lived in the village. Some days we had quite a social gathering at lunchtime as they all came in for a meal. We would have our Pat, Ann, Angie and Annie from over the road as well as Margaret, me and Ian if he was at home. Often two or three of the men would join us at the table if they were in the village at lunchtime. We didn't meet many people socially, so when we did we always enjoyed their company.

One night in the Spring we woke up to hear Ian moaning and screaming. We went in to see what was the matter. He was rolling around the bed, holding his stomach. When I managed to feel his stomach it was as tight as a drum, but as usual, Ian could not tell us what was wrong. After a while I rang Dr Cross, who came straight out at 3am. (This was when the doctors still did night calls.) As it turned out it was just a bad attack of indigestion, but Dr Cross was lovely about it. When we apologised for getting him out, he told us off and said we were never to worry about calling him out if we felt something was wrong. A lot of people complain about the Health Service, but we could not have had better treatment from our doctors for Ian if we'd paid for it. One thing is certain: no private medical insurance would have looked at Ian, so, like a lot of other people, we had a lot to thank the NHS for.

I went up north to buy a Vincent twin motorcycle and when I got home there was a pile of old Vincent club books with it. On the first one I picked up, the front page was black-edged in memory of a Bernard Cribb, a founder member and chairman. He had been killed in an accident on his Vincent black shadow in 1949. Living next door to us at that time was a Mrs Cribb, whose two children had the same names mentioned in the article about Bernard. So I went round and asked if he was her husband, and it turned out that he was. All the time that I had been messing about with my Vincents, she had never said a word about her husband and son riding Vincents.

Not long after this she became ill and it turned out to be cancer, we had met her daughter Diana but not her son Preston, who lives in Australia. Preston came home to see his mother and while she was in hospital he stayed with us. Mrs Cribb died a few weeks later and when the cottage came on the market Betty Barton, Ruth's mother, from Bishampton bought it. She only stayed about 18 months as she could not afford the £10 000 to get it rethatched, so she had to sell and move to Pershore. The young couple who bought it, Anthony & Jane Metcalf, were to become very good friends who shared our views about the environment and politics. Jane's brother David is handicapped, so she understood about Ian and was very good with him. They soon became like part of our family, which was good for Ian.

It was nice for Ian to have people coming and going, and it seemed that we always had someone or other here. Every year in Offenham we have Wakes week, which was always the last week in May. (They have now changed this date to the second week in June.) Different events take place all the week, ending on the Saturday with a church service and a parade down the main street. They close the street to traffic, and there are stalls down each side. The children and adults dance round the maypole that is 66 foot high and one of only five left in the country. There is usually a jazz band, the local brass band and acts like clog dancers. It was in 1985 that the WI asked us if they could do the teas from our house; ever since we have had a full house on Wake day. The only problem was that the Mencap Spring fete is always on the same

102

day as Offenham Wake, so I help in Evesham at the fete while Margaret helps the WI in Offenham. This is a bind as I miss the main day of the wake.

The Hells' Angels motor cycle chapter holds an annual event locally called the bulldog bash. That summer Julie and some members of the Bristol BSA motorcycle club went, and before going back home they called in to see us at lunchtime. Within an hour Margaret had a cooked dinner for nine on the table. She was always a great cook, and when anyone calls she will have a meal on the table before you can say 'Jack Robinson'. It is probably because we rarely went out that we were always pleased to have visitors, particularly for Ian's sake, as he got excited when anyone called. So everyone was welcome. It was a shame that Roy and Julie lived so far away as Ian got so excited when they came home for a few days.

We were hearing reports about a new home for the mentally handicapped that the health services were intending to build in Malvern. This was to have relief care facilities, so we were looking forward to getting more details, as there was always a dearth of places to enable carers to get a break. The place we had been using, Martin House in Dudley, was going downhill, and we had not been using it for some time. The Social Services were under pressure to provide accommodation and day care under the Care in the Community plan. Places like Lea Castle in Kidderminster and Lea Hospital in Bromsgrove were discharging their residents into the community. At the time there were no facilities for them to go to, so they had to build some. It was not too long before Social Services found this very expensive, so it was passed over to the private sector to find homes for the residents. Lea Hospital finally closed its doors for good: another facility gone for ever.

When we first moved to the Old Place I had trouble getting used to shop eggs. The milk we were buying looked like coloured water compared to our own Jersey milk and I hated the bacon. So I decided that at least we could still have our own hens. We had them for a few years before a fox got into the pen and killed the lot. At least we thought he had until a few weeks later we saw a hen in the garden. When I checked on the new hens we had bought, it became obvious that this was one that had escaped the fox. Then I found a clutch of eggs in the shrubbery, where she had set up home. We never did find out what she lived on for all that time, unless she was pinching the food we put out for the birds. When we put her back in the pen, the other chickens attacked her so we had to keep her loose in the garden. She began to think that she was one of the family and started to come into the house, which was quite amusing. It always surprised visitors when they saw her for the first time dozing on the kitchen floor with both dogs asleep a few feet away, totally ignoring her. She lived the rest of her life as one of the family. It's amazing just how long they live when allowed to see out their natural lifespan.

Ian had a passion for strawberries and raspberries so I had a fruit plot at the top of the garden by the chicken pen. We did have some very good crops but I noticed that we never had any on the bottom of the raspberry canes. One day I found out why. I went to pick some fruit for Ian's tea when I caught Pippen, our Stafford bull terrier, pinching all the berries she could reach.

I went to the French Vincent rally in Plomclin in Brittany. The French section always put on a great rally, which ends with a fantastic dinner. That year we had eight courses and a different wine with every course; you can guess what state we were in when we left to go back to the camp! Some of the more hardy souls then went to the local pub and were there till three or four in the morning. I won the award for the best Vincent Comet that year, due more to Jack Barker's efforts in rebuilding it than anything I had done. The plaque was too big and fragile to carry home on the bike, so Brian Werrett and his wife took it home in their car for me.

The mid-Glos sections of the of the Vincent club have always been keen on the French Rally. When we took Ian to the Glos rally near Slimbridge, we were always sure of a good reception. After the French rally Jack and I rode across France to look at some of the war cemeteries at Ypres and Tyne Cot. We booked in at a hotel in Ypres, then went to see the Last Post played at 7.30pm. They stop the traffic through the Menin Gate (which was built in

1927 as a war memorial) and play the Last Post, just as they have done every night since 1922, except during the war when they did it in the south of England. The 50 000 names on the walls of the Menin Gate, of Empire and Commonwealth soldiers who died and whose remains were never found, brings home the futility of war. It was a very moving experience; I don't think there was a dry eye among the visitors watching the ceremony. After spending the night in the town and visiting the museum the next day we headed out to the cemetery at Tyne Cot. This was another moving experience and made me think that all school children of 15 or 16 should have to visit these parts of France and Belgium to look at the results of the stupidity of war as part of their schooling. It seems that there is a cemetery off every street, sometimes two or three.

When I got back home I heard that they had now set the date for the opening of the special care unit. It was on 19 November 1985 that they finally had the official opening. It amazes me how the council top brass and councillors turn out for these occasions, totally forgetting how they blocked the project for years and giving the impression that it's through their efforts that the place is opening. It was a great improvement for the staff and clients of special care, not having to move around all the time and having their own space.

Ian was still only getting three days a week at the centre and having to go to Worcester for the other two days. So our next objective was to get him five days a week at Evesham. On the three days that he went to Evesham he took the mini bus. They began by just bringing him home and when he got used to the bus and escort, they collected him in the morning as well. The escort and driver on the bus were very caring and rarely get mentioned, yet they do an essential job, as they are the first contact in the morning. When they are kind and caring, as the ones who collected Ian always were, it made things so much easier for Ian and us.

Julie was swotting hard for her finals and doing her thesis for her degree. She had been talking about going around the world when she graduated. We said that we would pay for her ticket if she saved her spending money and worked while she was away. The only problem was that she was now having second thoughts about going as she had met Steve Campbell in Bristol. I said I thought that she should still go, and if he was really fond of her he would be waiting when she got back. So it was just after her birthday in March '86 that we took her to Heathrow to catch her plane. Her first stop was Greece, then Singapore for a few days. I rang a hotel there and booked her in as I didn't fancy my daughter roaming about Singapore at night looking for a room.

We had arranged for her to stop with Preston and Heather Cribb in Melbourne for a few days while she found her feet. Jack Barker had fixed up a job for her at a nature reserve called Arkarula in the Flinders mountain range in the outback. So after a few days of being shown the sights of Melbourne, she got on a coach for the long journey to Arkarula. We were quite proud of her travelling all that way on her own and meeting strangers. We were on tenterhooks waiting for her letters to arrive. She also sent her films home to save carrying them around so we could see the strange places she was visiting. One day the phone rang and it was Julie ringing from Australia. The nearest phone was over 100 miles away and she had got a lift on her day off. When she got there the telephone operators were on strike, so she got to talk to us for over an hour for the cost of a local call.

It really is a small world when you can talk over such a long distance. Another thing that proved this was when Julie went to a barbecue at work. Julie was talking to an English couple, and asked them where they came from. When they said 'Near Birmingham', she said she didn't live far from there, and where exactly was it. They said, 'You wouldn't know where it is, it's only a very small place called Dayhouse Bank.' Julie was amazed, and said, 'I was born there and my Granddad still lives there.' No matter where you go, you never know who is looking over your shoulder, so behave yourself!

CHAPTER SEVENTEEN

A t the end of March we attended another review of Ian's progress, or lack of it, at the day centre. Under general behaviour they made the following comments: *Ian's behaviour has been causing concern to us lately. He has become preoccupied with his own thoughts. He will often ask when Mrs Harbour is coming to fetch him.* (She was his escort on the bus and this was his way of asking when he could come home.) *He became very agitated when he could not have his own way, eg hold his book, car etc. Ian seems to have become a lot more withdrawn lately and is very rarely talkative and lively any more.*

Practical skills: Ian tends to be to be rather lazy if he can. he will not make very much effort to do anything if he can help it. He can now take his coat off unaided but is very reluctant to do so.

Motor skills & activities: Ian enjoys going for a walk and walks well, often at a pace. (This was because he often came out with me to take the dogs for a walk) *He enjoys swimming (for swimming read floating with help) and rides in the mini-bus.*

During the early part of 1986 we had got Len Young of Berry and Young, who were surveyors and architectural planners, to apply for planning permission. We wanted to convert the outhouse to provide a bathroom on the ground floor with access from the kitchen. It had been worrying us for some time that Ian was having to sleep upstairs, in case the cottage went on fire. We felt that we

107

would not be able to get him out of an upstairs window if necessary, as they were quite small. Ian would not understand the necessity of climbing through the window feet first. So we had installed him in the bedroom on the ground floor, the one I had built for Roy when we moved to Offenham, which meant having to take him upstairs to the bathroom. After looking around we decided that the best place was to the rear of the kitchen, as there was existing drainage in the outhouse. Len suggested we should apply for a grant towards the work as it was for the benefit of a handicapped person. We got planning permission and when the grant came through in July, I got Dave my bricklayer to start the construction.

When we cut through the kitchen wall we found that we had taken on quite a task as the stone wall was over three feet thick. Cutting through blue lias stone is a lot worse than brickwork but we got there in the end. I had decided to put a drain in the floor of the shower and toilet area. This meant that the whole room was a shower area. We tiled all the floor to drain to the outlet, with a shower seat bolted to the wall. This made it much easier to shower Ian, as we didn't have to do it in the confines of a cubicle. This layout impressed the grant people from the local council when they came to inspect the job, with the result that we got a lot of work doing the same type of conversion for handicapped people across the whole area. After a while a proper drain outlet was available commercially; up till then we had been using a standard bath drain outlet, which was not really suitable. This seemed to suggest that Ian's shower was one of the first of its type.

That summer we were avidly waiting for news of Julie's travels, and fighting to read her letters first. Later that summer I went with Jack to a German rally and he took me a roundabout way. We went to Portsmouth to catch the ferry to Le Havre, then across France to Chartres to see the rose window in the cathedral. We stopped there overnight and then went through Luxembourg and on to Germany. We went down the Rhine, which was quite a lovely ride. We then cut across Germany to the rally; when we got there we found that they were sleeping the visitors in the village hall. When we looked in there were sleeping bags over the floor, so we decided to find bed and breakfast in the village. As we don't speak German we asked one of the German members, who they called Willie Fixit for obvious reasons, if he could find us somewhere. He went round the local houses to find someone to put us up. He found a family quite close to the village hall who agreed to put us up. The only problem was that they didn't speak English.

On Saturday morning we came down to a huge breakfast. They gave us the key to the front door and then made us the same large breakfast on Sunday. When I tried to ask how much we owed them, as we were intending to leave on Monday morning, they got most upset and made it clear that they would not accept anything. So when we went to town I bought a large bunch of flowers for the lady of the house and some chocolates for the daughters. On the Monday morning they were all out but had left us breakfast and sandwiches for the trip. When I got home I wrote to them and got Margaret's brother John to translate the letter into German for me. It gives you a nice warm feeling when complete strangers can be so kind.

We were now eagerly awaiting the arrival of another grandchild. Our little Jenny was nearly five when Roy and Paula's second daughter, Emma, arrived on 27 December. We now had another lovely granddaughter to love. Ian was fascinated when he first saw her. He always liked his teddy bear and would carry it around with him. So it was a good job that he didn't think Emma was a doll or we would not have got her back!

Just before Christmas we had another review of Ian's progress. He was still not progressing much at the day centre and they suggested that he needed to go for five days a week if they were to make any headway with him. So we decided that he could go for the five days when the new enlarged special care unit opened after Christmas. I find it strange that only three or four years earlier they had told us that there was no call for special care in the area. Then before the new unit opened, they decided that it would not be big enough and they had to convert the old workshop into the new special care unit. Now, thirteen years later, after increasing the size yet again, the so-called Social Services are cutting the number of days that the clients can attend to three or four days a week to make way for new clients. So what happened to the lack of demand that they fobbed us off with just a few years earlier?

Roy had been off work sick for about three months with back trouble and early in January he had another medical. The Fire Service decided to retire him, because they thought he could put other members of his watch in danger if his back went again while on call at a fire. It's not until you know someone who is in the emergency services that you realise the rotten jobs they have to do. How many of us could carry a dying child out of a burning house, or cut dead or dying people out of the carnage of a motorway pile-up? And that's besides the danger they often have to put themselves in. Roy decided to apply for teacher training and got a place at Manchester University, so for the next few months until the course started he looked after the children while Paula went to work.

Julie got back from her travels in time to be with us for Christmas. After working at Arkarula, she travelled across Australia to Coopers Preedy to see the opal mines, on to Alice Springs and up to Darwin, before flying on to tour New Zealand, then spending a few days in America. Steve Campbell came to Heathrow with us to meet her. On the way home he told Julie that he had booked a trip to Finland to see some friends in March. Then he said they were going on his motorbike, a special with an off-the-road sidecar that he was having built by Pat French of Metisse in Bristol. After Christmas she went back to Bristol to collect her degree, then she settled in with Steve.

As the time came for their trip to Finland, they were having problems with the engine and took it up to Jack Barker's the day before they were due to leave. After working into the early hours, Jack sorted out the problems and they set off. After being in temperatures of over 100°F in Australia, Julie travelled across Finland with Steve in 30°F of frost. They were told by some Finns that they were crazy. It was so cold that when they cooked their veggi stew over a little petrol stove, they had to eat it while it was still on the heat. If they took it off, it froze before they could get it off the plate.

On the way back the bike broke down and they had to push it from Gothenburg to the ferry terminal, and missed the boat. They had to wait three days for the next one, with the terminal closed down till the next boat was due. They were lucky to find an open door to the ferry building, so they could at least wait in the warm, as they had no money left to get accommodation.

Steve had been doing up his house in Bristol and Julie was helping him. He also had a landscaping business and for a while they did some bed and breakfast. As they were vegans there was no meat served. After a while they started looking for somewhere in the country to live as they both wanted to move from the city. They were looking for a large property to do vegan bed and breakfast. I thought they were mad and that no one would go. How wrong can you get!

The much heralded residential home in Malvern was now finished. They named it Osborne Court and it consisted of four bungalows, each housing six or eight residents with their own day centre. Before they opened Osborne Court some bright spark (I could describe them differently but I don't like foul language) at the regional health authority proposed that they rent it to an insurance company. This caused a storm of protest and a lot of parents, including us, wrote to the health authority. Our first reply was dated 26 May 1987 and it went as follows:

Dear Mr & Mrs Wilkes

Thank you for your letter of 19 May 1987
I can well understand your concern regarding the long-term care of your son and have asked the Regional Medical Officer to look into the situation. He will be writing to you shortly.

T.A.Grosvenor
Head of Secretariat

Then on 5 June 1987 we received this letter:

Dear Mrs Wilkes

Mr Ackers, Chairman of the RHA, has asked me to reply to your letter of 19 May 1987.
Let me say at the outset that I fully appreciate the concern and worries you express in your letter about the long-term care of your son, Ian.

It went on in a long-winded way about how all the authorities acknowledged the need of handicapped people living in the community. They should try living and looking after someone like our Ian and a lot that are much worse; then we might believe their platitudes. He then went on to say that the Malvern unit would be opening shortly, with a similar unit being opened in Worcester in 1989/90, followed by a similar residential unit in Evesham to be constructed in 1991/2. It took two pages of waffle to say nothing at all. The Worcester and Evesham units were never more than a pipe dream. They have not constructed them and I doubt if they ever intended to or ever will. They have now privatised the home at Malvern. The letter was signed by Angus McGregor, Director of Planning/Regional Medical Officer. If he did know that his department was trying to rent it out to an insurance company, then he should have been honest about it, and if he didn't know then he was not doing his job.

Later in the year we had an interview at the Medical Research Council's project DIS-CO with reference to provisions for long-term care. Chris Bennett, the Research & Evaluation Officer, sent the transcript of our interview. It was rather a long and bitter tirade so I won't bore you with the full text but just give a general impression of what we said. For example, 'To this government, care in the community means privatisation'. Then I went on to point out that some private homes only want residents who can do jobs around the home and garden. (I know this from past experience). They don't want the ones who need a lot of looking after or are

112

disruptive. We asked them what would happen when we could no longer manage and were on our last bloody legs; would the only thing we could do be to take Ian with us? Such was the total lack of provision for long-term care then that you get to thinking that way, and it gets very depressing at times, it really does. Then we referred to the toy library that thousands of people had given money to and when everything was in place they said, 'You can't have anyone to staff it.' I then said that I got very angry with our area health authority, as the surrounding areas had much better facilities. If one area can do it, why not ours?

While all this was going on, many other things were happening of course. It was now becoming fairly obvious that we were never going to get any long-term care for Ian from either the health service or the Social Services. The health service was closing down places like Lea Hospital and Lea Castle. So when the secretary of our local Mencap branch, Daphne English (who has been the driving force behind the local Mencap since its inception, and still is) said we should be looking for another project to raise money for, the committee discussed several projects and finally decided to try and build another home for the more handicapped residents. The local society had opened one some years earlier called Brook House, and the new home was to be for the more severely handicapped.

When we started we were hoping to house four residents, but it soon became obvious that this would not be economically viable, and we would require a minimum of six. We decided that we would need a steering committee, so Daphne talked a local accountant, Bob Bailey, into joining us, who in turn persuaded another local person, Ann Albright. They became essential members of the committee. I was also on the committee but mainly to make the numbers up, I think, at least until we got down to the building work, which was when my building experience would become useful. I suppose I had an ulterior motive as we were desperate to get Ian settled in a home we approved of before we became too old to look after him. We had heard horror stories of Social Services finding places for handicapped people out of county when their

113

carers were no longer able to cope. This compounds the problem, as the carers are unable to see their loved ones.

As well as raising funds, we approached Wychavon District Council to see if they had a site that they would give or lease to us for the new home. Their reaction surprised us, as they were very helpful. As well as offering us a site, they offered to prepare the drawings, which would save us money. They had done the same a few years before for Brook House. It was the start of a long process, as it was to be several years before we opened the home.

As all this was going on, I was making arrangements for my motorbike trip to the continent. The Vincent Club were holding an international rally in Europe in 1987 and we intended to attend. I booked my ferries and was looking forward to meeting a lot of new people. They were going to hold it in three parts over three weeks, starting in France, then Germany and the final week in Holland. Jack was club social secretary so I was keeping up to date on what was happening. The club was bringing Phil Irving and his wife from Australia. Phil had helped to design the Vincent motorbikes, in conjunction with Phil Vincent, in the 1940s. Also coming were Burns and Wright who had broken the world speed record in the 1950s on a Vincent motorcycle on the old tramway in Christchurch, New Zealand. They took both solo and sidecar records. At the Dutch part of the rally, two world famous bikes would be there, Mighty Mouse and Super Nero, and both were going to be run on the road near the rally site.

CHAPTER EIGHTEEN

Ian was spending five days a week at the day centre now but from time to time the staff had a training day, which meant that Ian was at home on those days. Margaret made a habit of taking him out to town for a walk and calling in at a cafe for his cup of tea. Then, as always, she'd buy him a little car or other small toy.

One Monday I went with them and while I was in the library, Ian had a very bad fit in the street. People were so good: some shop keepers came out and one of the taxi drivers wanted to use his radio to get an ambulance. By the time I arrived Margaret had it all under control, and all I had to do was wait till Ian started to recover and get the car. There never seemed to be any warning when Ian was going to have a fit, even when we were watching him. When the chips are down there are a lot of very nice and helpful people about. I also think that a lot of the people who look the other way or cross the street to avoid you are not rude or intolerant, just embarrassed. Or maybe they think that the person who has had a fit or is drunk.

I set off that summer to go to the French rally, which they had arranged so people could go on to the German section of the International rally. A group of riders from overseas were to meet at Jack's house in Dursley, so he could act as guide. I had arranged to meet them there. There were members from America and New Zealand; among them I met John Hugot and Marty Dickinson from the States, who were to become friends. They still visit us when they are in the UK.

We set off for Portsmouth to get the ferry to Le Havre, then on to Plomeun in Brittany. We had a great time there, including the section dinner of course, and when the rest set off for Germany, I came home on my own. I could not leave the business for three weeks as I had some tenders to finalise. We had arranged some relief care for Ian for the week after I got back, as Margaret and I were going to the Dutch section of the Rally. Julie and Steve were also going on my spare bike. They set off the day before us as they were staying with friends near London.

The following morning, when we were due to start, it was pouring with rain, and when you have a ferry to catch you have to go no matter what the weather. I thought that Margaret would get soaked before we got very far, so I rang the coach company to find what time the London coach went. By the time we got to Evesham the coach had left so I made a dash for Broadway and caught it there. To kick the Vincent over to start it, you have to lift the passenger foot rest. In the rush we forgot to put it down and Margaret put her foot on the hot exhaust pipe. The result was a very badly burnt shoe. Margaret had bought them new to go away in, so she had to travel all the way to Dover hobbling on a shoe with the sole burnt away.

I had got very wet by the time I arrived in Dover so I found a B & B and booked a room for Margaret and me. Next morning the weather had improved, and we met Julie and Steve in the queue for the ferry. When we got off in France we set off and stopped for a meal in Belgium. Julie and Steve asked for vegetable soup, so you can imagine Steve's reaction when he found a piece of meat in his. On the continent it would appear that they think a vegan is someone from outer space! I took it back and exchanged it for some chips. I thought it best not to ask what they cooked the chips in, even if I could make them understand.

We stopped overnight on the Dutch coast at a farm that had a caravan for hire. Julie and Steve pitched their tent and after dinner the heavens opened, so they moved in with us for the night. It was a lovely ride next day as the weather had improved and we rode past miles, or should I say kilometres, of deserted beaches. We were making for the rally site that was just outside Delft. Margaret and I had booked into a hotel and Julie and Steve were camping at the rally site. The Dutch section had got a full week of events for us. We went to see the flower auctions which they hold every day: it is a huge place, so large that employees have to ride round the building on little motorbikes.

Another day we spent at the Dutch police headquarters. They escorted about 200 Vincent motorbikes from all round the world to the police headquarters, even stopping the traffic on the motorway to let us on. The chief officer welcomed us in four languages and they laid on a four-course meal for over 300 people, and entertained us for several hours. We spent a day in Delft, then later in the week, the police stopped all traffic on one of the local roads so Super Nero and Mighty Mouse were able to run. (I am sorry to say that I find it hard to imagine our police being so helpful; they would have been 20 or 30 years ago, but not now). It was quite a spectacle and the noise was deafening. On the last day the Dutch section had baked a huge cake dotted with all the national flags of the different nationalities at the rally. I think there were members from over 20 countries there. We all had a fine time, and it was nice to have Margaret with me at a rally for a change.

We got home and one of the first things we did was to collect Ian. They said that he had been fine, but we knew he had missed us and that he had been worried because once again his psoriasis was so much worse, particularly in his hair - what he had left of it, poor lamb. One of the things we had been trying to do for several years was to get better advice about Ian's epileptic fits. Pearl Barker suggested that she could contact the David Lewis Centre for Epilepsy. In their reply they said that Ian would have to go for at least 12 weeks, possibly extending to 26 weeks, if they agreed to take him. We thought it would be too traumatic for him and decided against it. Whether we made the right decision or not, we will never know. It is just another thing to fret about now, when we try to figure out why Ian died.

We were told that Osbourne House in Malvern was now open for relief care. They had decided that, as they had employed five senior staff, they would have to find something for them to do until such time as they came to a final decision about the future of the building. They were still considering renting it to an insurance company. So we decided to book Ian in for an occasional but regular overnight stay, to see if he could get used to being away from home. It was in early in 1988 that we were to get our first opportunity for relief care, such was the demand. We booked Ian in for one or two nights at weekends about every six weeks for the next year, mainly to get him accustomed to being away from us as part of our build-up to finding a home for him

Meanwhile, in the latter part of 1987, Julie and Steve started looking in Scotland for their new home. They used to go up on the train and as they had a dog they would come up to stay overnight and leave the dog with us before going on to Scotland. Hippy was a large Alsatian bitch, but such a gentle thing and she got on well with our dogs. I used to take her and Pippin, our Staffordshire, with me when I went round the jobs. I had to leave Toby at home as he would wander off if I did not watch him.

We were doing a job at a school in Redditch during the half term and I had to leave my car in the street as we dug up the drive at the school. As I was walking back to my car, a crowd of youths were hanging about filling the pavement, and showing no sign of moving aside to let me through. Hippy and Pippin were still round the corner with the lads. I whistled to them and as they came rushing up to me, it was like the parting of the Red Sea as the whole crowd of youths scattered.

We were having Hippy quite often so I said they should leave her with us until they found somewhere in Scotland. The first place that interested them was a castle on the coast at Stonehaven, so they asked me to go up and have a look at it. I drove up and took Jack Barker with me to share the driving. (As it turned out he drove most of the way.) Although the present owners had modernised one wing of the castle, I thought there was too much work to do on the rest of it to make it a viable place for them. It was the sort of place I would have loved to buy if I'd won the pools and could afford to do it all up. Not that that was very likely, as we very rarely did them.

Steve had been doing landscape gardening in Bristol and when he was clearing out the ground, where he grew trees and scrubs, he brought them up to Bishampton to plant on our land. We purchased 1500 whips (this is what they call very small trees) to plant with them. So when they arrived, Julie and Steve got a crowd from the Friends of the Earth in Bristol to come up for the weekend and help plant all the trees. We used over 20 varieties of British broad leaf trees, and all our helpers slept in the barn on straw. As most of them were vegetarians, Margaret had cooked a load of veggie stew in the old copper, the one that we used to cook the pig food in. It's a good job they didn't ask what we had used it for. She did clean it out first, just in case you wondered! It was a great weekend as several of them brought their musical instruments, and we had a sing-song round a camp fire. Without their help we would have taken weeks to do the work, Thanks, guys and girls.

The steering committee for the new Mencap home was now meeting on a regular basis and Bob Bailey was finding sources of funds. Wychavon Council's architect department was doing a splendid job of the designs for us to consider. One was a wonderful layout all on one floor. As usual we had to make some compromises. In this case it was the amount of land the design would take up, so we had to go for a two-storey building. I thought that we would require more recreational space, so we asked them to design a room on the side as a garden room. This we felt needed to be part of the original design, so it would not look out of place if we added it on at a later stage.

We did not think that we would be able to afford it when we started to build the home. We were fortunate in that we had a very generous, anonymous donation of £15 000. This was worth £20 000 if you took the tax rebate into account. This allowed us to build the garden room at the same time as the rest of the building. Work on site was not due to start until early in 1993 due to the various problems we encountered. Even after Wychavon Council allocated the land to us, problems kept arising. Worcestershire County Council insisted we would have to construct a roundabout to provide access to the site. We were to be the first building to be constructed in a new road, which was a blessing in a way. It meant that we would not get the usual objections against putting a home in an area of existing houses.

The arguments about the road entrance were to drag on for over two years. Then Wychavon decided to sell off their housing stock to a housing association. This meant getting the existing tenants to approve the transfer, then the council decided to form their own housing societies, one to cover the Droitwich area and one for Evesham and Pershore. As you can imagine, all this took time. Then council decided that they would not have any use for an architects' department now, as they did not have any housing. So all the work that remained on the project was given to a private architect.

To avoid further delays with the construction of the new road and housing that our project was to be part of, Wychavon passed it over to an existing housing association called Bromford Carinthia. This changed the whole basis on which we were to work. Instead of us building and owning the home, we would have to pay rent for the building. This had advantages for us. First we would not have to raise so much money and the rent was reasonable, as we were providing for a social need. But the financial commitment was still huge. We had to equip and furnish eight bedrooms, six for the residents and two for staff, as well as the other accommodation, and pay for what we had originally thought of as a garden room. They had scaled down the building size to bring it to budget. If we had not paid for the extra room it would not have been big enough to reach the standards required by Hereford and Worcester Council Social Services Registration Department. The council would not have allowed it to open. It seems a bit strange that no-one, neither the architect or Bromford Carinthia, had the foresight to realise that. With all the problems, construction did not start on site until early in 1993.

That was all in the future so now back to 1988. Ian loved going to the pictures and the local cinemas were very good, never charging for him. They always saved a seat at the back if they knew we were going, as Ian rocked from side to side all the time we were in the cinema. One time we went, as usual we waited till most of the people had moved towards the exit before getting up to leave. As we stood up Ian was violently sick. I went to the manager and asked for some cleaning materials, explaining what had happened. He would not let me do it and told me not to worry, they would clean it up. Life in general would be so much better if there were more people like him about.

Ian certainly had no modesty. To give one example: we had joined the Green Party after going to a talk at Malvern by Jonathan Porritt. Although we had been lifelong socialists, we liked the agenda of the Green Party. At one meeting in St Andrews church hall in Pershore, Ian kept letting out noisy, ripping farts, and saying in a loud voice: 'Ian let Polly out of prison'. He thought it was very funny and would laugh loudly every time he farted. No one took any notice and totally ignored it, but when the smell got too much we had to take him to the toilet. The only one big enough to get him into and attend to him was the ladies, so Margaret had to take him in while I stood guard to stop any ladies from going in. Even someone like Ian, who is quite capable of walking, still needs the use of a handicapped toilet. We had to help him undress and we clean him up after he had been to the toilet. If a handicapped toilet is not available it can cause problems. They keep most handicapped toilets locked and you have to travel quite a distance to get a key. There is a scheme whereby you can buy a key that fits a lot of toilets in most parts of the country, but unfortunately not all. Even on motorway stops you have to go to the office or shop to get a key.

That year I decided to go to the Vincent rally in Sweden and as no one I knew was going, I went on my own. I rode to Harwich, took the ferry to G'o'tborg then rode across Sweden to the Baltic Sea. The rally was taking place inside the Arctic Circle so we were hoping to see the midnight sun but for me it was not to be. I was just heading north towards the Arctic Highway when I came to a roundabout. As I went round it I met a car head on coming the other way. It all happened so fast that I have never been sure who was going the wrong way, the car or me. I had to get a breakdown truck to take the bike to a garage to get it patched up.

121

It so happened that he was on his way back to G'o'tborg so he took me all the way, and only charged me for part of the way.

When I got a hotel I rang Margaret and told her the bike had broken down and I would get the next boat home. I had just missed one ferry so I had to wait four days for the next boat. I at least had time to explore some of Sweden, including travelling up the coast by boat, even if I was stiff and sore. They have boats travelling along the coast calling at all the islands like water buses, so you can stop off, look around and catch the next boat a couple of hours later or stay overnight. Although Sweden is very expensive, most of the people speak English so that makes travelling easy. But I couldn't figure out was what was wrong with most of the people I saw. Then after a few days I saw someone smile and I realised that he was the first person I had seen smile. So I now knew what was wrong.

When I got back to Harwich I had a long ride home. I had a problem with the luggage rack; it kept falling off and I had to stop and tie my bits and pieces back on with odd bits of string. I spent over 12 hours on the road getting home, then got a telling off from Margaret when I told her what had really happened for not telling her at the time. At least she was glad I was still in one piece.

CHAPTER NINETEEN

Julie and Steve were still looking for property in Scotland. They had seen one they liked at a price they could afford in Ballater in the Cairngorm Mountains. Jack and I took another trip up north to look it over; I thought it was quite sound and knew that Steve was capable of doing the work that he would have to do. So they decided to buy and moved in during September, hoping to be ready for the Christmas trade at their vegan guest house. Ballater and the surrounding countryside was very impressive. A river ran just by their house and, walking over a bridge, we saw some small wild deer in the meadow, drinking out of the river. You could see the large red deer higher up on the mountain. It amused Jack and me that a lot of local shops had several large coats of arms with 'by appointment' engraved on them, just a reminder that Balmoral Castle was just up the road

Roy and Paula decided they needed a larger house now that they had the two girls, so they also bought a new house and moved in during November. With Roy starting a new career and moving house, it was all change for him, Paula and the children. Ian was, as usual, very happy when we told him we were going to see Roy and the family in their new house. We could never tell Ian what we were going to do the day before the event, as he always expected to go immediately and didn't understand he had to wait. So we soon learned to tell him what we were going to do at the last minute. It made life easier for us and less stressful for Ian.

Christmas that year meant a lot of travelling. We stopped off at Roy and Paula's new house to leave the Christmas presents, then did the long drive up to Ballater. We stayed there a couple of days before heading home to spend Christmas. We always felt better at home with Ian in case he was off-colour, as he often was at Christmas, probably due to all the excitement. Then we were off to Roy's for Emma's birthday on the 27th. Ian was OK to travel that year, but it was not always the case. Some years we were not able to go as Ian was not well enough. A handicapped person causes problems for the whole family, not just the parents. It's difficult telling a small child that her grandparents can't come to her birthday, when we were promising to go right up to the last day. Jenny and Emma were always very good and accepted it quite well.

It was in January that the day centre started to run a home-teaching scheme. The idea was that Charles Waring, who was now Ian's key worker, would bring Ian home at lunchtime and get him to prepare his own lunch. This was more hope than anything else, I think, because all the time it went on Ian never progressed very far. At least they were trying to help him, and I have to give them full marks it for it. Basically the idea was that Margaret would keep up the training when she learned the procedure. I think you try anything to improve the standard of life for your loved ones, but I always had a gut feeling we were not going to get very far. There were small improvements so it was not a waste of time. To have succeeded to any greater extent a lot of work would have had to be done when Ian was much younger, not 32, as he now was.

Even with Charles bringing Ian home there was still trouble, as Ian had one of his rare fits of temper and hit out at Charles. So they decided that Ian would have to have an escort to come home with him and Charles. As there were no resources available, they asked Margaret to go to the centre, bring Ian and Charles home and take them back after lunch. This went on for a few months until they stopped the scheme. The special care unit had grown quite a lot and the number of staff increased, with Ann now in charge, as Sue had left when she had twins.

The first overnight stay for Ian at Osbourne Court in Malvern came early in January. We had taken him a couple of times for an hour each time and stayed with him, so the staff could get to know him and it would not worry Ian too much when we took him to stay overnight. Even so, he was quite apprehensive when we got there, as he had always hated change and I am sure he could read our minds or at least sense our worries. We always felt guilty when we left him and were wondering how we would cope when he went to the new home. In some ways we thought it might be better, as the carers in the home would not change as frequently as they seemed to in relief care. It seemed to us that every time we took Ian to the relief care accommodation, there were different staff members to brief about his drugs and his behaviour.

In some ways we were glad of all the delays in constructing the new home. At least it put off the day we were dreading, when we would have to bite the bullet and take Ian to his new home. We had a walk round the shops in Malvern before collecting him on the Saturday lunchtime. The only thing Ian wanted to do whenever we collected him after a night away was to go straight home. The staff said that he had not been any trouble, but then they always said that. I must say we never had any reason to complain about the care Ian received at Osbourne Court; the staff were always very kind and caring.

We were still using Cross Roads to look after Ian while we had an evening out, and between them and Osbourne Court, for the last part of the eighties we had a greatly enhanced lifestyle. Only someone who has experienced living with a handicapped or elderly person will know what it feels like to look out of the window on a lovely Spring day and say, 'Let's take the dogs for a nice long walk along the river', then come down to earth with a bump and say, 'No, you go, I'll stay and look after Ian.' It seems such a tragedy that it is always 'a lack of funds' that restricts so many necessary benefits to the more vulnerable in our society. It never fails to amaze me how quickly our government can find the money to buy arms and fight wars, often just hanging on America's coat tails.

Margaret had been keeping a diary to record the frequency of

Ian's fits. Looking back at this diary now, I see that he was having between 12 and 30 fits a month. In 1989 his daily drug intake was as follows:

8am: 2no 500mg Epilim, 1no 200mg Tegretol, 1no 5mg Folic Acid
4.30pm: 1no 500mg Epilim, 1no 200mg Tegretol, 1no 5mg Folic Acid
10pm: 2no 500mg Epilim, 1no 200mg Tegretol, 1no Frislum

This was a daily total of 2500mg of Epilim and 600mg of Tegretol. Any more drugs and he was like a zombie, any less and the number of fits soared. He was also on Steroid cream and ointment, and Betnovate scalp treatment for his psoriasis.

In February we took Ian to Manchester to see Roy and family. Ian was all excited when he saw Roy, especially when Roy took him to the shops to buy him a matchbox car. But he had his usual reaction when we were back home on the Sunday and had three *grand mal* fits one after the other, so he spent most of the day asleep on the sofa. It's so sad that nearly every time he was happy he had to pay for it by being unwell.

The following week Jack and I went to the German Winter rally again, so Margaret had to cope with Ian on her own for the week, including taking him to the dentist. He always enjoyed the attention, calling the dentist 'the doctor' and his assistant 'the nurse'. The following Saturday Pat Hill met Margaret in Evesham to help her with Ian and give her some company. On the Sunday Margaret took Ian and the dogs for a walk, and said in Ian's diary that she wouldn't do it again in a hurry. So I assume she had some problems with three dogs and Ian as well. Ann would have Ian in the office for the odd hour to give Margaret time to take the dogs for a walk, and Ian always enjoyed having someone else to fuss round him. Meanwhile, Jack and I started back from Germany in a snow storm, which made life interesting. While I enjoyed going away on my bike I was always happy to get back home.

Ian had another weekend at Malvern in March. Then the following weekend we went to see Margaret's brother Vic and his wife Edna. All the way there Ian worried that we were taking him back to Malvern, repeating all the time, 'Betty (his escort from the

126

day centre) bring Ian home' and 'Don't let the nurse put Ian to bed'. So although everyone told us that Ian had been OK while he was away, this was the sort of thing that told us he really was uptight when he was away from home. Even though it was upsetting us as well as Ian, we felt that we had to persevere with it to try and get him used to it, to ease the trauma we knew it would cause all of us when he moved to the new home.

The day centre proposed taking Ian away on holiday, as the more able in the main centre went every year. We thought this was a good idea, and said we could always fetch him home if they had any problems. They left on the Sunday afternoon and returned on the following Friday. Ian seemed quite happy and the carers who went with the group said he had enjoyed it. The difference from Malvern was that on holiday they were going out every day, having snacks and drinks while out, often in pubs, which would please Ian.

One of the things that he enjoyed at the centre was going swimming, well, really lying in the water with his water wings on and someone supporting him. He would come home and say, 'Ian been swinnin' but then he always did like a bath. Most days Margaret would give him a shower; once or twice a week she would give him a bath, but only if I was about in case he had a fit there. He was now over fourteen stones, so it was virtually impossible for us to get him out of the bath on our own, without a lift. We did think about fitting a lift, but it was not possible with the low ceilings in our cottage.

When Roy came down with the family, Ian had a lovely time, especially watching the girls playing. When they were babies he loved to hear them cry, jumping up and down saying, 'Baby cry'.

Just after my birthday Ian had a series of fits, so many that we sent for the doctor. It turned out that he had a high temperature, which is a common cause for fitting. It was after this that the doctor gave us a prescription for rectal Valium, which was a godsend, as in the past Ian had to have an injection of Valium. They injected it in the muscle so the doctor had to do it, and it always caused Ian a great deal of pain. Now we could insert the pessary when he had a lot of fits in a short time. This meant that in a few minutes he was out cold for several hours, waking up much better.

Margaret was still going for her check-ups every six months, to make sure that she had no recurrence of her breast cancer. She never seemed to worry about it, or at least never showed it. Ever since Ian had been going to the day centre, Margaret had been writing a diary every weekend for Ian to take with him on the Monday, and they would fill in what he had been doing each day. They could then talk to Ian about the things he had done at home, and we could talk about what had been going on at the centre. Not only was it useful at the time, but it is invaluable now when I am trying to tell his life story.

I often went for a ride on my motorbike on a Sunday morning if the weather was nice. I would usually start out about six in the morning, taking a bacon and egg sandwich and a flask of coffee, then riding over the Cotswolds or over to Wales and stopping to have my breakfast on some common or wild part of the countryside. The best thing about going so early was that there was very little traffic on the country lanes. Also I could be home by the time Ian was awake and help Margaret get him showered and dressed. We are so lucky to live in a lovely part of the country, where I could get to remote areas without going very far on main roads. Eating your breakfast early in the morning in the countryside, miles from anywhere, with no sounds other than the birds singing is one of life's little pleasures that everyone should try. If Ian woke up before I got home he would get excited, constantly saying, 'Daddy gone on motorbike', so he got a lot of pleasure too.

When I went to the mid-Gloucestershire sections Rally at Slimbridge, I would go on my bike and Margaret would bring Ian in the car. The mid-Glos members always made Ian welcome, especially Vera and Brian, for which we will always be grateful.

One of the bigger contracts I had on the books was a new village hall at Sedgeberrow. We had finished it that summer and the committee invited Margaret and me to the official opening. We took Ian with us and all the men who worked on the job also had invitations. It's always nice when people appreciate the work we do, and say so. I was lucky to have such a good work force; we had built up a good team, including our sub-contractors. I always used the same ones unless the architect nominated other contractors. I found that if you look after your staff and sub-contractors, they will always help you out when the chips are down.

CHAPTER TWENTY

Besides the fits that Ian suffered from during the night, he had now also started to get up in the early hours to go into the kitchen. The first time he did this, we were amazed at how he had managed to get into the kitchen with no lights on, even getting past the three dogs without disturbing them. It did not happen very often, but we thought we would leave a couple of low lights on so he would not hurt himself when he wandered about in the night. We had always left a night light on in his bedroom, so he would not be worried if he woke up in the night; he wasn't able to switch a light on himself.

Early one morning we heard Ian laughing fit to bust. When we got down to his room he was sitting on his bed, ripping the lightshade (one of those pretty paper ones) to shreds. We had only bought it a few weeks earlier, thinking he would like a colourful shade with pictures on it, but perhaps he didn't. We usually heard him moving about in the night and that was more important than us not hearing him, even if we were losing a lot of sleep; at least we knew he was not coming to any harm.

Ian had some funny ways. If you asked what he'd had for dinner he would say something like 'Aunt Margot's got sore nails'. Then a couple of hours later he would say, completely of the blue, 'Ian like fish and chips' so you finally got your answer about what he'd had for dinner. If he got upset with me he would say, 'Daddy go to the office, or go to meeting'. When he got upset with Margaret he would tell her to go to the WI or shopping.

130

We decided we would like to go to stay with Julie and Steve for a few days and Roy said, 'Why don't you leave Ian with us in Manchester and have a break?' It was in the school holidays; Roy could look after Ian full-time and the girls liked making a fuss of him so we knew he would be OK. We took Ian to Roy's and stopped overnight, then carried on to Julie's the next day. We rang Roy each night to make sure Ian was all right. We had a lovely time cycling around the lovely country lanes. Margaret went on the tandem with Steve, and I had a job to keep up with them, as they did more cycling than Margaret and me.

Then on the third night when we rang Roy he said that Ian had had a bad fit in the night. The intensity of the fit shocked him, and he said fits like that would kill Ian one day. We assured him that people do not die from epilepsy. Time was to prove us sadly wrong. Roy said he could still look after Ian and asked us to stay with Julie. We decided to go home as we felt Ian would feel more comfortable in his own surroundings. I always think you are better at home when you are feeling poorly.

When we had been back from Scotland a few weeks I set off for the FIM rally in Barcelona. The Vincent Club were trying to get a lot of Vincents at the rally to see if they could get the award for the biggest single-make club at the rally. (In the end we came second to the BMW club.) I met Jack and we rode down to Portsmouth to get the ferry. I always liked waiting for the ferry because we usually went to the front of the queue. They put the motorcycles on first, and you tend to meet other bikers from all over the place. A South London section member had planned the route that we would all take, with the lunch and overnight stops set out so that, although we went in small groups at our own pace, we could all meet up at the arranged stops.

We travelled south through France and up onto the high roads of the Pyrenees. We then went through Andorra and on over the border into Spain. We travelled on down to Barcelona, and followed the signs to the rally assembly point. After we booked in, local members of the FIM on scooters guided us to our hotel on the Las Ramblas. The receptionist told us we would have to find safe parking, because if the police didn't book us, we would only find the chains that we had locked the bikes up with by morning. When we did find an underground garage, we had to pay the same as the cars - about £15 a night, although you could park four bikes to each car space.

We did have a lovely time there and the final event at the rally, was a parade round Barcelona. There were over 2000 bikes at the rally, from all over Europe. A lot of the riders tied their national flags on the back of their bikes on tent poles, so it was quite spectacular. It was so hot most of us rode round the route in shorts and tee-shirts. Motor cyclists do not have to wear helmets in the city, so we went without. The next day I set off for home on my own. The rest of the Vincent Club were riding back along the south coast of France, and I was catching the ferry from Santander to Portsmouth. I stopped overnight on the way and when I got there I found I had two days to wait.

When I finally got to Portsmouth, Customs stopped me and had I to empty all my luggage out. By the time I had unpacked it was dark and my lights gave out. So I was riding round Pompy with no lights and having the usual problem of being turned away from B & Bs because I was in biking gear, although at 62 I would have thought people would realise I was not a trouble maker, and my bike was worth more than most of their cars. This is something I have never found on the continent. I have even stopped in four-star hotels while touring on my bike. I did finally find a place and had an uneventful ride home the next day. Although I had enjoyed the break I was happy to be home.

As Julie was going to be busy in the guest house for Christmas and the New Year, we decided to go and take up the Christmas presents early in December. As we were taking Ian, we went in the motor caravan. It was an old one with a lift-up roof, but we thought that Ian could lie down or draw while we were travelling. All went well until we were going up Shap Fell on the motorway, then the roof blew up and Margaret ended up hanging onto it to stop it blowing away. I had to creep along so Margaret could hold it down until we reached Carlisle, where I turned off into the town.

We found a chandler, purchased a long length of rope and tied the roof of the camper back on as best we could. After a slow journey, including several stops to check the roof was still there, we finally made it to Ballater, exhausted.

The next day I went to the local hardware shop for some self tap screws. I said that I had better have a selection as I wasn't sure what size I needed. The shopkeeper asked what I wanted them for and I told him what had happened, so he said, 'Take the box and bring back what you don't use.' I did the job and when I took the box of screws back I asked him to charge me for 20 of the largest size as I had used different sizes. He would not let me pay, as he reckoned I had enough problems. It sort of restores your faith in humanity when people are so kind

After a few days we set off back home and as we stopped for breakfast at a service area just outside Glasgow, we saw someone trying to hitch a ride. I asked him where he was going and when he said 'Down to the M5', we offered him a ride. We found that he was going to Cornwall so we were able to give him a good start. He turned out to be a busker and entertained Ian all the way down, playing his guitar and singing. When we stopped again to get some food, he said he would wait in the caravan. After we had talked to him for a time, we found that he was broke so we treated him to a meal. Later, when we dropped him on the M5, Margaret slipped a fiver in his pocket as a way of saying thanks for the time he'd spent occupying Ian.

A little closer to Christmas we went to Roy's to see the girls and take their presents. We always went up again the day after Boxing Day for Emma's birthday. This year was the exception, as both Ian and I had very bad flu-like colds. We were both ill and not fit to travel so we missed Emma's birthday that year. I always feel sorry for children who have their birthday near Christmas, as they always seem to be missing out. Perhaps the parents should have arranged it better!

We had not been able to go and see my father in hospital over Christmas because of the colds Ian and I had, so it was early in January before we got to see him. He had gone into the hospital in

Redditch with pneumonia. I thought it was a disgusting place, as it never seemed clean to me. You could feel your feet sticking to the floor when you walked down the ward and some of the equipment was dirty. This was in total contrast with Ronkswood Hospital in Worcester, which in spite of being an old wartime temporary hospital, was always sparkling clean in our experience. While Dad was in hospital they decided he would not be able to look after himself for a few weeks, so the Social Services arranged for him to go to a retirement home in Bromsgrove for a few weeks. He was now 88 and after a few weeks in the Broom House, he decided to stay on a permanent basis. He thought it was great having everything done for him.

We finally got to go to Roy's early in January. The weather was terrible, raining all the way there and back, and I hate driving in bad weather on the motorway. Our next door neighbours, Anthony and Jane, were always very kind to Ian, inviting us to any parties they had and making a fuss of Ian. His odd behaviour never worried them; if he had a fit, they just took it in their stride, as did all their families. It was the same in the local shop and post office. Carol would often give Ian a comic when Margaret went in with him. He would get so excited when someone other than Margaret or I gave him anything. When other people made a fuss of Ian it would tug at our heartstrings.

At the end of January we had a postcard from Julie. She started off by saying that they were having a break in a lovely place overlooking the Isle of Skye. Then she went on to say that we should sit down as she had some news for us. She said that they had got married that weekend. I had always said we would get a phone call one day to say they had got married. At least I nearly got it right! It appears that you can take out a marriage licence anywhere in Scotland, then get married somewhere else, as long as it is in Scotland.

A few days later we had been showing the postcard to someone who called to see us, and must have left it on the kitchen unit. That night we were woken up at about 4am by Ian laughing, when we got down we found him sat in the kitchen, a pile of paper at his

134

feet. He had found Julie's postcard on the work top and torn it into very small pieces, much too small to try to put together again. How he managed to find things in the dark I will never know, but he did. After that episode I thought that I had better do something about it, so I had a sort around in the workshop and found a micro switch. I screwed it on the door frame and wired it to a battery and a bell in our bedroom. It worked a treat and every time Ian got up in the night we heard him via the bell. Not that it worried us, him ripping things up, but it did worry us that he might pick up a knife or some other thing that he could hurt himself with.

Julie came down for two weeks on 14 February. I took Ian with me to meet her off the train at Cheltenham, and he got so excited when I told him where we were going. It was a shame that he was going away on holiday with Charles from the day centre on the Tuesday, but he would have plenty of time with Julie when he got back on the Saturday. Steve flew down from Aberdeen on the Sunday and we picked him up at Birmingham Airport. Ian went to Devon for his short holiday and was so pleased when he got home and found Julie still here.

While Julie and Steve were here they decided to have a party for their friends, as they lived so far away they didn't see them too often. The following weekend, about 20 of them turned up and most of them stayed overnight. Roy and family also came down for the weekend, so we had quite a crowd, so many that we had to put some up in a couple of tents on the lawn. Ian was quite bewildered by it all but enjoyed himself. He loved to watch Jenny and Emma playing, and luckily he didn't have any fits till everyone had gone home. Roy left on the Sunday evening, and Julie on the Monday morning, so from having the whole family around us for a change, we were soon back to our normal routine. Margaret had a few tears when we said goodbye and they all went home, as the house felt empty. It seems that excitement comes in small doses. I suppose that it's the same for most people: if you stop to analyse it, life slips by in a routine way, with highs and lows only coming from time to time.

Most weekends we tried to take Ian out for a meal and to the pub for a drink and a packet of crisps. Eating out was one of the things he enjoyed most. I suppose it was the wrong to do as he was overweight, but I am glad we did.

Whether it was a reaction to all the excitement of the last few weeks or not, I don't know, but we had been having a few problems with Ian. He went potty in the car on the way to Bromsgrove one day, and we had to stop the car, as he got very distressed. He was shouting, 'No bath road' and throwing himself about in the back of the car. Both of us had to hold him tightly until he calmed down. We were not able to find any reason for these outbursts, because at other times he was OK.

For a few weeks we were living on tenterhooks, never knowing when the next outburst would come, often in the most embarrassing places. The public will overlook a young child having a tantrum or just mutter to themselves about it. When a 34-year old man has a tantrum like a child, you get some funny looks and comments. Looking through Ian's diary I saw that one morning Margaret had sent a note to Charles at the day centre. It read: 'Ian was up early this morning and he's like a time bomb; hope he's OK today'. Then after a few weeks he calmed down and things were back to normal, at least normal as we know it. We will never know if he was in pain or suffering in some other way, poor lamb.

The trees we had planted had suffered in the drought that summer: we had lost two or three hundred. As we came to the end of the summer we were keeping a close eye on them so we could order all the replacements we needed for planting during the winter. The old mobile home we had put on site was a godsend, as Margaret could make Ian's cups of tea and do some food. Ian could draw and be amused in comfort while I was working on the land. We still had the three dogs and Hippy was still following Ian around everywhere he went.

CHAPTER TWENTY-ONE

The previous year I had seen a sports sidecar I liked at the Motorcycle Show at the NEC in Birmingham, so I ordered one. They fitted it to my Vincent for me and we tried to get Ian to go in it. After a while he started to enjoy going out on the sidecar. The only problem was getting him out of it, which was a bit of a struggle. After a few trips he got the hang of it and managed better. Our first trip was a bit hairy, as I had not ridden an outfit for 30 years and had forgotten that when you take a left-hand corner, the sidecar comes off the ground. On our first trip I took the sharp left-hand bend out of the village and couldn't get round it, so we went right over on the wrong side of the road. It nearly put Margaret off going on it again, but I managed to persuade her to try again.

We had some nice trips, including taking Ian to some of the club rallies. I was using my special for my solo trips, so I was getting the best of both worlds. One of our first trips was to the mid-Gloucestershire section of the Vincent Clubs rally. They hold it every year near Slimbridge, the wildfowl sanctuary, so it was not too far to take Ian. We always had a warm welcome, with Vera and Brian making a fuss of Ian, though we were never able to camp out with Ian so we only went for the day.

Early in the summer Ian went on another holiday from the day centre, or training week, as they called it. The idea was to encourage the clients to do more for themselves. I think it was an uphill struggle with Ian, but I do admire the patience of all the staff. I don't think I could do it - it's different with one of your own children but someone else's kids are another ball game. When they came home the staff always said that Ian had had a good time and enjoyed himself. They thought we didn't believe them, and as they took a video camera to record some of their activities, they showed us how well Ian had settled, which was nice. The staff also made a video of the activities at the centre, which was quite an eye-opener to us. Ian always complained about going to the centre, and very often played up when we were trying to get him ready to go. So the staff took a video of him going into the centre and he ran in laughing. He was just trying it on with us, so we didn't feel so guilty about sending him after that, though he still tried it on.

I went to the French rally that summer, and I took the ferry from Plymouth to Roscof in Brittany. As usual the French section put on a good rally, and when I got back we went to see Roy and family in Manchester. Ian always loved going to see them and was very good all the time. The wheelchair we had for Ian folded up so we could put it in the back of the car. While Ian could walk OK, he got distressed if we went too far, or if he had been having some fits. When he had a series of fits in the night he would be lethargic most of the next day; it was times like this that we needed the wheelchair. It was also useful to keep in the car so it was handy if he had a fit while we were out.

The bell I had rigged up to let us know if Ian was up and about during the night was working well. He seemed to be up and about during the night about every couple of weeks or so now, but we could get to him before he got into the kitchen. We usually made him a cup of tea and sat with him for anything up to an hour before he settled and went back to bed. Then, in between, he would have three or four fits in the night, we never required an alarm to let us know when he was fitting, as he used to make a lot of noise. It's amazing how quickly you react when things like that happen during the night. If you hear the phone ringing at 3am, it takes ages to respond and it's stopped before you get there.

During the school summer holidays we would meet Roy and Paula on the motorway and bring Jenny and Emma home for a couple of weeks. The company was good for Ian as he enjoyed watching them play, and thought it extremely funny if one of them had a little tantrum. I had built a large swing in the garden and Ian also had a trampoline, so the girls had some fun on them, and it got Ian outside as well. I think they looked on Ian as a large doll, because they liked helping to dress him and getting him things. It didn't seem to bother them when he had a fit or when he had a strop, as he did from time to time.

Early in August Margaret went to stay with Julie for a week, so we had booked Ian in to stay at Malvern, as I was very busy at work. We always had plenty to do during the school holidays, as we did a lot of maintenance on school buildings, in both Worcestershire and Warwickshire. This meant we were all working six and seven days a week, trying to get all the work cleared up. The day centre had agreed that Ian could come to the centre every day from Malvern, so it wouldn't be too big a break from his usual routine and hopefully he would settle better. Margaret went by train to Aberdeen, and Julie collected her from there to take her to Ballater.

While Margaret was away Ian had one of his bad fits during the night. They tried to ring me from Malvern the next morning but I was out, so they rang Margaret in Ballater, which shows how worried they were at the severity of the fit. Ian often had ones like during the night but no one believed us. After I collected Margaret from the station we went straight to Malvern to collect Ian. He got so excited seeing us that he held Margaret's hand all the way home.

The summer of 1990 was long and hot, or at least that is how I remember it, so I had plenty of use out of my motorbikes. I often went to site meetings on my bike and got some funny looks when I walked into the meeting with a crowd of suits and ties. In leathers and helmet, pony-tail and a big gold earring, I stood out like a sore thumb. Still, they soon got used to it and it probably got us more work in the long run, because I was an odd one out and they remembered me when tenders were going out.

In September I set off for the continent again. I was sailing from Plymouth and as I was just going into Plymouth my bike lost all compression. I rang the RAC and when the man arrived he took one look at the bike and said, 'What's wrong? You probably know more about this bike than I do'. So I told him I thought the piston had a hole in it. He thought I was right and arranged to transport the bike and me back to Offenham. So bang went my holiday. When I stripped the engine I found a small hole in the piston, as clean as if someone had drilled a hole in it. After talking it over with Jack, we came to the conclusion that when I'd fitted a new carburettor, I had damaged the gasket and it had been sucking air. This had caused it to run on too lean a mixture, resulting in the piston damage. I always did learn my lessons the hard way.

Ian came home one day from the day centre with a kitchen roll holder that he had made in the workshop. He was so happy when he gave it to his mom, saying 'Ian made this'. I think that a member of staff had done the turning, but they assured us that Ian had sanded it down, varnished it and assembled it. No matter, it still holds pride of place in the our kitchen and we are proud of it. The day centre did not close for long holidays in the summer like schools, but only for two weeks, like most industrial firms. This year Ian had only been back a couple of weeks when we decided to go up to see Julie at Ballater, very much a spur of the moment decision. After our problems earlier with the motor caravan roof, we decided to sell it and buy a Range Rover, as we thought Ian could sleep on the back seat if he got tired. So this was a chance to try it out. We stopped the first night at Roy's and then carried on to Julie's the next day. We had a lovely few days there and on the way back we drove home in the day, nearly 500 miles. Usually we were exhausted when we arrived home after driving back in one day, but after driving the Range Rover back, it was amazing how fresh we were when we got home. Of all the vehicles that we have had over the years - and that includes a BMW - the only one I would have again if money was no problem would he another Range Rover.

A couple of weeks after we got back, I collected the post and when Margaret opened the one addressed to Ian she had a shock. When she showed me the letter I went ballistic. It was from the

DHS, saying 'Do not cash any more of your disability allowance and return your book at once. Legal action may be taken against you'. About three weeks earlier a doctor had called to see Ian. He was retired, and the DHS use retired doctors to do home visits and assess whether the handicapped person is still entitled to the allowance. On this occasion Ian had a good day and responded in some small measure to the doctor. I think this doctor must have had a brain storm as he obviously reported that Ian was not handicapped. For two weeks I rang the DHS in Liverpool several times a day, but the person who sent the letter was never available. After a couple of days I wrote, and when I had not had a reply I wrote every day. After three weeks I was still very angry, so I went to see our local MP, Michael Spicer. When I showed him the letter I said that I wanted the benefit reinstated and the person responsible for the fiasco sacked. I explained that Ian had not been able to go to the day centre for years as they said he was too difficult, and was only able to go when the special care unit opened. I told him to so speak to our doctor and community nurse.

Michael Spicer must have acted pretty fast as within two weeks we had a letter of apology and they restored Ian's benefit. I never found out if they sacked the civil servant or whether he just had his knuckles rapped, but I would bet he never had a dickey bird said to him. I then said to Margaret that she should apply for attendance allowance. We had never bothered to apply for it before, but I thought: if they can act like that we will get everything going. We also applied for the mobility allowance for Ian but it took 12 months and a change in the law before we got it for him. I still get angry when I see so many people with not a thing wrong with them getting all the benefits going, and boasting about it as well. Then, to cap it all, when Margaret turned 60 they said that she was not entitled to a pension, as she had no stamps. Had she drawn attendance allowance all those years she would have got one. So my advice is make sure you get all the benefits you can lay your hands on.

About twice a year the dentist came to the day centre in a travelling surgery. This time he said that Ian had got a decayed tooth that had to come out. It was bad on the side, so he couldn't fill it and if he didn't

141

extract it Ian would have trouble with the adjoining teeth. He suggested we take him to the NHS dental unit in Worcester so he could remove it there. He didn't want to do it at the day centre, as it might put Ian off going to have them checked in future if he got frightened.

Ian got excited when we told him we were going to take him to see 'the doctor', as he called the dentist. We set off for the clinic in Worcester, and found that the dentist was a lovely man. He asked if we wanted to stop with Ian while he removed the tooth. I am a bit squeamish, so I was not too keen but Margaret said she would. I thought I had better stop as well so I didn't appear too much of a wimp. As it happened, there were no problems, When the dentist told Ian to open his mouth for the injection, he did. While we waited for the injection to work, Ian rocked to and fro in the chair, very happy. Then the dentist said, 'Open your mouth, Ian' and he opened it wide. The dentist only appeared to look inside Ian's mouth, and when he turned round, I asked if the tooth was going to be much trouble to get out. He said, 'Not really, here it is'. He had taken it out so fast we could not believe it and I don't think Ian had even noticed! He was still very excited about it all, enjoying all the attention.

I was thinking of putting a wood burning stove in the dining room, but when I opened up the back of the inglenook the stonework was so bad I had to rebuild it. So I spent the next two weeks sorting stone from the garden and rebuilding the back of the inglenook. I got Dave in to help me put the stainless steel chimney liner in and Geoff to plaster the ceiling we fitted to the inglenook to stop the drafts in the room, then I fitted a villager log burner. It had much more character than the gas fire we had used when we stopped using the open fire. With the thick thatch, small windows, the insulation and secondary glazing I had fitted over the years, the cottage needed little heating, so we could just use the stove in very cold weather. At first we did have some fires and sat there sweating just to get the effect.

I still had a very good crew working for me and the business was doing well. We were getting more work than we could handle at times, which is almost as bad as not having enough, or so it seems when you are struggling to get it done. Well, you have to have something to worry about, don't you? Roy and family came down to stay at the end of the summer holidays. When Roy played Margaret's guitar and sang to Ian, he would rock back and forth, singing in time but putting his own words to the tune. He still liked me to play the keyboard to him, but didn't get as excited as when Roy played for him. Perhaps it was because I was not very good, at least nothing like as good as Roy.

CHAPTER TWENTY-TWO

In the October of 1990 I saw a coach trip to Holland advertised in our local paper. I noticed that one of the tours was to a little village just over the border in Germany called Monshau. Jack and I had called there coming back from the German rally some years earlier, and I had promised Margaret I would take her there one day. It was all a bit of a rush as we had to make sure we could get Ian a place at Malvern for the five days we would be away before we could book it. Luckily, Osbourne House had a vacancy.

We stayed in a nice hotel in Valkinberg, Holland, and spent the first day looking around, which was quite nice. On the second day we set off to Germany for a trip down the Rhine, to the Renaegn Bridge, which had been made famous in the film about the American advance into Germany. Then it was off to Monshau, but when we got there I was a bit disappointed. Although the village was much the same as when I first went, they had changed it for the tourists. Whereas we had ridden right down into the village on our first visit, there was now a car and coach park at the top of the hill and you had to walk down into the town. They have also built a cafe and restaurant adjoining the car park, making it all very commercial. When you come across somewhere out of the blue, it appears more enchanting. Still, I was glad that I had taken Margaret there, at least she had seen somewhere that I talked about when I came home from my trips.

Just after we got back, Roy and family came down for the weekend, which pleased Ian, especially when Roy gave him a shower. Little Emma helped Roy, she was like a little nurse with Ian, always doing things for him. He always liked having someone running around waiting on him (a bit like me, I suppose!)

Most weekends we tried to get Ian out and about, visiting the different towns in our part of the Cotswolds. One day in early November Margaret took him into Evesham and they met Pat there. During the conversation they talked about the Christmas presents. Ian was on to it like a flash and talked about Father Christmas for the next seven weeks, singing jingle bells all the time, which got a little tiresome in the end.

With Ian's psoriasis getting worse, there were times when we could not shave him as his face was so sore. It was also in his hair and on a lot of his arms, legs and body, so in desperation we started to take him to an alternative health centre in Southampton. The doctor held an electrical device like a magic wand and passed it over Ian. Then he clipped wires to Ian's toes and fingers and took readings on an electric meter. He said Ian was allergic to dairy products, tea, coffee, chocolate and cheese, also anything with beef or rice. We found it quite alarming and were wondering what we could feed him. They also gave us several bottles of medicine - at a cost, I might add. If my memory serves me correctly, we were paying £40 a visit and another £10-£12 for the medicine. We went every month for over a year before coming to the conclusion that it was not making one whit of difference. So we called it a day. Perhaps we should have realised much earlier that it was a waste of time, but when it's your own flesh and blood you try anything.

The steering committee for the new home was still meeting on a regular basic and trying to raise more money. The local Mencap Society always had a party just before Christmas for all the local people with learning difficulties, and as usual they all spoiled Ian rotten. A few days before the party we had a snow storm that cut off the village and we were without electricity for the weekend. As we have log fires and the Aga is gas fired, we were quite comfortable. The only difficulty was taking Ian to the toilet by torchlight. We also had some paraffin lamps, but I had a job to find any paraffin until the next day, when I emptied some out of the greenhouse heater. So we were OK for the remainder of the weekend, and did some cooking for the neighbours who were all electric, so had no heat or light. Ian thought it was funny and enjoyed himself enormously.

We had arranged to go to see Roy and the family on 17 December, but Roy rang to say that it was very foggy and the forecast was not very good, so we put the trip off till Sunday. On the Saturday we went to buy Ian some slippers and he had a bad fit in the shop. I went to get the wheelchair from the car, he was still poorly when I got back and the assistant had to help get him into the chair. Ian slept most of the way to Roy's the next day, but when we got there he brightened up. We had a good Christmas with Ian, he was quite cheerful all the holiday, and he even opened all his own presents for a change. What with all the visiting we were doing and people who coming to see us, we had a busy and one of the best Christmases we have had for a long time.

One good bit of news was that Ian was at last losing a bit of weight. In the last month he has come down from 15 stone 11 to 15 stone 3, which was a nice surprise.

We seemed to be having a lot of visitors in those days. People were turning up most weekends. At times two or three couples would arrive on the same afternoon or evening, which was nice for all of us, especially Ian. We were still taking him to Malvern every six weeks for an overnight stay, hoping to get him used to being away from us. It wasn't working too well, so we were getting worried as the date for him to leave home was getting closer. However, Ian seemed to be getting a little bit brighter. He queried your answers when you responded to his questions. The down side was that when he went to bed he would lie there laughing fit to bust till the early hours. While it was nice that he was having a brighter spell, it got a bit wearing when he kept us awake till two or three in the morning, especially when I had an early business meeting, often half an hour's drive away. I would arrive looking like something that the cat had dragged in.

We had started some restoration work at Pebworth Church. Dave was doing the exterior stonework and Duncan and one of the apprentices were replacing the floors internally. One of the jobs was to reposition a very old carved oak screen to make way for an organ to be installed. When we fitted it in the new position, we found that it was two feet short. I gave them a price to make a new section to match. When we had made and fitted it, it looked as if it had always been there. Doing work like that gives me so much pleasure, and makes me realise how lucky I am to have spent my life doing what I like and getting paid for it.

We had Jenny and Emma during the half term in March, and Roy came down for a couple of days. When they went back, we went down to Southampton to see the doctor again, as there was still no improvement in Ian's skin condition. Good Friday was on 5 April and on the Saturday we took Ian and Pat to Ludlow for the day. Ian always enjoyed it when we had company on our trips; I think he got tired of only having his mom and dad around him most of the time. We called at a cafe called D'Greys and they had the best toasted teacakes I have ever eaten, they were scrumptious. Ian was still going through a bright stage, chattering a lot more and pointing at things like pictures on the wall and kitchen cupboards, and asking, 'What's that?' It was as if he had been in a coma for years and was just emerging.

Margaret is a natural optimist and I am pessimistic, so she said he was getting better, while I tended to look on the black side and think about when he would revert to his autistic ways. So between us we tended to steer an even course, rather like Jack Sprat and his wife. She ate all the fat and he ate all the lean, so they licked the plate clean.

Sometimes when Ian came home from the day centre, he would wander up to the office and Ann would make him a cup of tea. He always enjoyed someone else doing things for him and when I was doing things around the house or in the garden, he loved 'helping Daddy'. One Saturday when we were in Evesham we met Ian's escort, Val. When we met her Ian said, 'Ian don't go to the centre', which, silly as it seems, pleased us because it was another sign of how he was improving. It meant that he not only recognised Val, but associated her with the day centre. When you have a child like Ian it's amazing how such small things can give so much pleasure.

The next weekend Ian had a very nasty fit, so on the Saturday when we went to the Vincent rally in Gloucester, we went in the car so Ian could sleep on the way. Although Vera and the others made a fuss of Ian, they got little response as he was in a daze all day. He hardly noticed what he was eating when we had our picnic, which was most unusual for Ian. The local Mencap were still running the music club one night a month in Evesham. Ian loved it, as did most of the other members. The local people who give up their time to play and sing to them deserve a pat on the back for their sterling efforts.

Towards the end of May, Ian had gone on holiday with the day centre again, and while he was away we collected Julie and Steve from the station at Cheltenham. When Ian came home on the Friday he was so surprised and excited to see Julie, he had a very nasty fit. The following weekend we were back to normal as Julie and Steve had gone home. On the bank Holiday Monday I was on the gate taking the entrance money at Red Gables. The house has lovely gardens which the owners open to the public three or four times a year in aid of charity, in this case Brook House. Margaret brought Ian up in the afternoon and they had tea and cakes.

The weather has not been so good that year, so I had not been using the bike as much I would have liked. Later in June we had been promising to take Ian to the seaside for a day out, but on the Saturday it was pouring with rain. Ian kept saying, 'Ian's a seaside boy', so we didn't have much option and off we went to Weston-super-Mare. As Margaret said later in Ian's diary, 'The weather was so bad it was plain crazy to go'. Yet Ian enjoyed himself, laughing all the way, and when we got there we didn't have any of his usual 'Ian don't like rain'. We had fish and chips for dinner and then went for a walk down the pier and had some ring doughnuts. No wonder Ian was over fourteen stones! At least we had the foresight to take some dry clothes with us. We took Ian into the handicapped toilets to change him: not that it mattered, we could have changed in the road and no one would have noticed, as the rain was still belting down and the place was deserted.

At the day centre Charles had been off work for some weeks with a bad back, and Ian was showing signs of missing him. One of the problems with autistic people is that they dislike any change in routine, and it showed.

It was the end of June before the weather improved, and on the spur of the moment we decided to go and see Julie and Steve. It all depended on being able to get Ian into Osbourne Court for a few days. As luck would have it they had a cancellation in a couple of weeks. We had just enough time to make arrangements for the transport to take Ian to the day centre and back to Malvern every day.

CHAPTER TWENTY-THREE

While we were away the staff at Osbourne Court kept a brief diary of what Ian was doing there. On the first day, the comments were as follows: *Day 1 - Ian arrived at Osbourne Court mid-morning and settled well, but got a little perturbed when a female client got over friendly towards him. He made several attempts to kick her away, but we calmed him down and he has been fine since. Day 2 - Ian has eaten a good breakfast but we were not able to shave him as his face is too sore. We have applied locoid cream and will try tomorrow.* Days three, four and five had just one line of comments about how well Ian had eaten, then on the sixth and final day, Ian suffered a *grand mal* fit at 6.30am and made a slow recovery. Most of the entries were very short; we had hoped for more detail, similar to the diary that Margaret and the day centre filled in every week.

We had a very pleasant week with Julie. The weather was lovely and on the way there we took the secondary roads instead of going on the motorway. Julie had some good news for us: she was expecting a baby. Margaret was overjoyed, but worried because they lived so far away. Julie was a wonderful cook but as their guest house was strictly vegan, I used to eat at the hotel on the other side of the road where they did lovely 'carnivore' food. Until, that is, they started cooking and serving only Indian food - then I had to find somewhere else to eat. Someone from Oxfam must have once stopped with Julie and Steve, because Julie received a letter from them out of the blue asking if she would do some of her recipes in a section of their Christmas book. So that year all our friends had an Oxfam book for their Christmas present. It had some nice photos of the prepared food and also a nice picture of Julie. We came back the fast way and got back in the late evening. The next afternoon, when the escort brought Ian home, he dashed in very excited and so pleased to be home.

At the end of July, Roy had to go to a summer school at Stirling as part of an Open University maths degree he was doing, so as Paula was working we had the girls for the week. Not that it was any hardship as we loved having them, and it was good for Ian to have them around. We took them all out in the motor caravan (we had by now got a larger one). We had picnics and went out rather more than we usually did, including taking them to Mrs Bomford's for riding lessons, so Ian enjoyed that too. The thing he enjoyed most was when they squabbled, as sisters do, and one of them would squeal at the other. Ian would jump up and down, laughing fit to burst. Roy came to stay for a few days before taking the girls home. I set off for the French rally a couple of days before he arrived, so Margaret had a couple of hectic days looking after them all.

To add to Ian's problems he had been suffering from bad piles for some time, but at last we had some cream that seemed to help. At least it stopped the bleeding.

We were due to go to a vintage bike rally with Peggy and Norman, but just before we set out Ian had a bad fit so we couldn't go. Ian tended to sleep for several hours after a bad fit and the hot weather we had for most of that summer made him have more fits than he would normally. This was a shame as it was nice to have such a good summer for a change, especially for bikers!

The following weekend we met Pat in town and went for a cup of tea, then she came home with us for the afternoon. It was a good job we came home because when we walked round Evesham with Pat we did not get far, as every other person knew her and wanted to stop for a chat. Ian loved her company and liked to hear her chattering on. The next day we went to see my Aunt Dora in Leamington, who Ian had a real soft spot for. He was always talking about his Aunt Dora, but strangely enough he would be exceptionally quiet when he was with her, partly, I suspect, because she never stopped talking!

Colin and Doreen from Bradford came to stay for a week at the end of August. The day centre was closed while they were here and Margaret was worn out by the time Ian went back, and our visitors had gone home poor. I wasn't much help as we were always busy finishing off our school jobs in time for the start of the new term. Jane and Anthony were always regular visitors, dropping in several times a week. Once we told them all about when Ian was small, nearly making their hair stand on end at some of his antics. We had plenty to laugh about as well so it made an interesting evening.

Our Mencap trip that year was to the Severn Valley Railway. We went to Bewdley by coach and caught the train to Bridgenorth. It was so hot and Ian was uncomfortable so we just found a pleasant pub and stayed there till it was time to go back. The next week Roy and the family came down for the weekend. We didn't go far and had a late night round at Jane and Anthony's, as they had a barbecue. Next morning Jenny and Emma went wild doing some cooking in the kitchen, which fascinated Ian. When they said goodbye, he wanted to get in the car and go with them. He seemed to be experiencing more feelings that year, getting more involved and showing less autistic tendencies that we had noticed in previous years.

Ian still enjoyed music. He didn't mind my feeble attempts on the electric organ, and enjoyed Margaret playing the guitar, especially if she sang as well. She has a nice singing voice, so I enjoyed it too. The monthly music club run by Mencap was still going strong. Ian enjoyed these evenings out, but would get in a tizzy if we did not sit by him.

Margaret was now doing some shopping for baby clothes, and knitting like mad ready for when Julie's baby arrived. Margaret's brother Vic had found an old cine film with Ian, Roy and Julie on and I had it transferred to video, although there was only about ten minutes of film. It so impressed me that I thought we should get a video camera so we could get record our grandchildren's childhood. Charles was now back at the centre as Ian's key worker after several months off, so Ian was now back into his routine.

One evening in October we took Ian out for a bar meal. When we were halfway through Pat and Graham came in, and Ian shot up from the table and rushed to greet Pat. It always threw him when we met someone he knew well in an 'unusual' place, as he always expected to see people where we normally saw them.

One Saturday night in the middle of October we came down in the morning and, as usual, we went in to see how Ian was. We found him sitting on the floor by the bed, fast asleep. We hadn't heard a thing in the night so we don't know what happened. He seemed bright enough so we didn't think that he'd had a fit in the night, as he was always lethargic for hours after having one. In fact, he was quite the opposite for the rest of the day, and kept asking, 'Who's Richard's mother?' or Guy's mother, or anyone he thought of. He even asked his granddad, not that he ever understood what Ian was on about anyway. Much as we loved Ian, his behaviour could be a bit wearing.

In the office I had taken on someone to help Ann. Sandra fitted in like one of the family, and was a great help. When Ann was on holiday Margaret had to look after the office in the afternoon as Sandra only worked mornings. Ian always seemed to know he had to be quiet while she was on the phone. On the odd occasions that he was a bit vocal, our suppliers and clients understood, as most of them knew Ian.

One night when we were watching the main news on BBC we got the shock of our lives to see Julie and Steve walking down the main street in Stonehaven. Julie was very pregnant and looking a bit self-conscious about it. Steve was the Green Party Parliamentary candidate for that part of Aberdeenshire and a reporter was interviewing him about his policies.

Now that the nights were drawing in and getting colder, we tended to spend more time by the log fire in the evenings. I would make some bread and then play the organ, or Margaret would play the guitar and sing to Ian. Sometimes Anthony and Jane would pop round and this

153

would keep Ian entertained. For some reason Ian would call Jane 'Ruth', no matter how often we told him it was Jane. We went to see my dad on his birthday; he was 90 in November. He still gets about OK and goes into the town for a walkabout most days.

Ian's fits were getting steadily worse, and someone asked who his neurologist was. We said he didn't have one, and it amazed them that Ian hand never been referred to one. They said we should get the doctor to refer him to a specialist. We got an appointment for Ian to see a Dr Betts at the Queen Elizabeth hospital in Birmingham on 18 December. Ian had a very bad fit in the street in Evesham just before we saw the specialist and once again people were extremely kind. We were keen to find out if the doctor had anything to offer that might help Ian. He was still going to Malvern for an overnight stay every six weeks, and Margaret took full advantage of the break to get some Christmas shopping in.

The following Wednesday we took Ian to see Dr Betts for his second appointment, and after a lot of discussion he decided to add a fairly new drug called Lamictal to the other drugs Ian was taking. After a couple of days, we got quite worried as Ian started to have a series of *petit mal* fits. He was having as many as 10 or 12 an hour, as well as some funny shaking turns. We rang the hospital to speak to Dr Betts, who didn't seem particularly worried and just told us to give Ian half the daily Lamictal intake for a few days and see what happened. We felt that the doctor should have given us some warning of the possibility of this occurring. Things did quieten down after a while, but it was scary for a couple of days.

We had a quiet but very pleasant Christmas, with lots of visiting. It's amazing just how long it takes to do the rounds of relatives and friends. Still, it cheered Ian up as he had not been well, having had a couple of fits on the Saturday. There was still no news from Scotland about our newest grandchild; probably Julie did not want to part with it! Then, early in the morning of 7 January we had a phone call from Steve to say that Julie had just given birth to a little boy - well, not so little really. He weighed in at nine pounds, three and a half ounces. Then Julie came on the phone to talk to us. She'd had a bad time and they had rushed her to the Aberdeen

Hospital during the night. She told us that they were going to keep her in for a few days. It upset Margaret that she had not been there with Julie, so I got on the phone to Birmingham Airport and booked her on the first plane to Aberdeen the next morning. She was going to catch the last plane back the same day, which meant she could see Julie and the baby for a few hours. It meant an early start and late return, but Ian barely seemed to notice that his mum wasn't there, mainly because he was at the centre all day. It amused Ian that I was cooking his tea, and he kept saying, 'Whose daddy is a mummy?' Our new grandson's name is Karma Rune Campbell, which I thought was a bit of a mouthful at the time, but it's surprising how quickly you get used to it.

CHAPTER TWENTY-FOUR

In the middle of January 1992, Margaret went to help Julie for a few days and took Jenny with her. Julie was trying to get the house ready for the guests who had booked in for the end of January, but she really wasn't fit enough after the rough time she'd had having Karma. Not that Margaret was as much help as she would have liked, as she went down with a very heavy cold. Like Julie, she did too much when neither of them was fit, so it was not as happy a time as she would have liked. Still, life is like that. Ian was happy to see Margaret when we went to collect her from Birmingham Airport, especially when Roy turned up to collect Jenny.

Not long after Margaret got home we watched a programme on TV about house insulation, and the area they chose was Balliter, where Julie lived. They said the reason for going there was that it is the coldest town in the UK. Margaret said, 'I can well believe it after staying there in January'.

One day I was looking at a job we had to do at the day centre when I bumped into Ian just as he was going to lunch. It surprised him to see me there, but I think he was more interested in getting his lunch to take much notice of me. It was nice in a way, as not too long ago he would have wanted to come home with me. We had Roy's girls for a few days during the half term, and they came with us when we took Ian for an EEG at Kidderminster. It impressed them when they saw Ian with lots of wires stuck on his head. The funny thing was that his results were normal, and they said that he

156

might have to have a mobile unit that he could wear for 24 hours. I could see us having to sit up with him to stop him taking it off, even while he was asleep. In the end it didn't come to that as when they repeated the EEG a few weeks later, they had much better results.

At the end of that week Julie and Steve also came down with Karma and invited a load of their friends to a party to meet him. It was an exciting time for Ian to have everyone he loved around him and a lot of other people as well, with plenty of music and food. To Ian that was heaven on earth. When we were on our own again, Ian went back to having a nap in the afternoon, but didn't like us saying that he had been asleep.

One evening our chimney went on fire. While we were in the lounge with a nice log fire, I noticed a roaring noise and went outside to look up at the chimney. When I got outside I saw several people watching the flames coming out of the chimney. Alan from over the road came over and said that he had rung the fire brigade. A few minutes later they arrived and soon sized up the situation. They were marvellous, even putting down runners to protect the carpet when they came in. It amazed me that they made no mess, and carefully cleaned up as they came out. At least Ian enjoyed all the excitement, with the pumps roaring and all the firemen dashing around. The good part was that there was no damage at all, due to the efforts of our local fire service. We couldn't thank them enough. They told us that if we had any trouble in the future, we had to be sure and tell them that it was a thatched cottage. When all the excitement had died down, you would not have known anything had happened. I think their prompt arrival and professional approach says a lot for our local fire service.

I had seen a BMW motorbike for sale that I fancied, so we had a trip out to see it. Margaret drove home while I rode the bike - needless to say, I bought it! I was not using the bikes much during the winter but I was looking forward to my early Sunday trips. I still intended to use my Vincents abroad and the BMW for a quick blast around locally at the weekends. Ian loved going out in the sidecar, so I would often take him to see his granddad in it.

Easter was now here and we decided to have a picnic on

our land at Bishampton to check on how the trees were doing. The following weekend the weather was lovely on the Sunday so we decided to go to Weston on the spur of the moment. I never like travelling on Bank Holidays, I find it better to go before or after, when there are not too many people about and we can park on the beach for the day. Luckily Ian had not had any fits all day, which made a change, as he had been having a lot of minor fits or absences lately. These were quite weird; when he went into one of these fits the right side of his face or right arm twitched and he dropped anything he was holding, though he was quite unaware of having dropped anything. He had so many of these fits at that time that Margaret rang Dr Betts' secretary at the Queen Elizabeth, who said she would ring us back after she had spoken to the doctor. The only suggestion was to reduce the number of new tablets. Perhaps we expected too much but we thought they should have examined Ian, and his reaction to the new tablets.

Roy and the family came down for a long weekend, and Ian followed Roy around everywhere. It was as if he couldn't get close enough to him. After the weekend we booked Ian into Osbourne House at Malvern for a few days. We then decided to go up to Scotland to see Julie and Karma - a long trip but worth the effort to see our Karma again. I was lucky that I could leave the running of the business to Ann in the office, while Geoff ran the jobs. When we got home the staff at Malvern said that he had been good, but he was glad to be home. He kept saying, 'Ian don't go Malvern today'. He seemed more lively, not wanting to sit around so much, which was lovely but very wearing for Margaret, who as always bore the brunt of it.

The spring holiday was quite a busy time as there was the usual celebrations round the maypole for Mayday in the village. On the Saturday we went to Manchester for the day and I looked after Ian, Jenny and Emma while Margaret and Paula went to see Roy get his maths degree from the open university. He wanted the extra degree, as he decided to specialise in teaching maths. Margaret had been dying to see Roy in his cap and gown, and she

158

got a lot of pleasure from her day out. After a wet start to May, by the middle of the month the weather had improved and we were thinking that summer had arrived.

I was looking around the camping shops to find a tent to take on my motorbike to France in a few weeks' time. The one I had was too small for comfort and I wanted something larger. I eventually found what I was looking for, a two-man tent that opened like an umbrella and was small enough to carry on the bike. As usual while we were out and about we stopped for a meal at a pub. We knew we would never get Ian's weight down like this but what the hell, he enjoyed it so much. When we got home Ian got upset and cried, saying he wanted to Roy to come and see him. It brought a lump to our throats. He so rarely cried that when he did we felt like crying with him.

One of the things Roy taught Ian was how to catch a ball and Ian proved to be quite good at it. The only thing was, as with most of the things he did, he soon got bored with it, saying, 'Ian's done that'. We were still taking him to the music club every month and he really loved going. He would stand and rock back and forth if it was his type of music. He had very definite ideas of what music he liked.

The weather was so hot that we were staying at home during the day and taking Ian out for a drink in the evenings. That is the advantage of living in a thatched cottage: they are cool in the summer and warm in the winter. It was even too hot to go out on the motorbike, so I was not going very far afield during the day. We are never satisfied, are we? In the winter we want the summer, then it's too hot.

We had another appointment with Dr Betts about Ian's fits. He wanted us to increase his new tablets by half a tablet every morning, but not until he had written to our GP. We were still worrying about the severity of the fits, as sometimes after a bad fit Ian would hold his head, moaning with pain. We would spend the next hour or so putting wet tea towels on his head, which we had put in the fridge to cool down. None of the medical people seemed to believe us when we told them how bad it was, which was quite frustrating.

Our friends were now commenting on how much Ian's vocabulary had improved. It could be a little embarrassing when someone who didn't know Ian very well called, as most of our friends always brought something for Ian when they came. A little toy, comic or just the magazine from the Sunday paper, it didn't matter to Ian what it was as long as they gave him something. When someone called without giving him a little present, he would ask where it was. In the end we kept some of his little cars by the front door for people to give him when they came - silly really, but anything for a quiet life.

Early in July Ian went on holiday to Devon with the day centre to stay in a cottage for five days. There were four staff and four clients, so with the weather being so nice they were able to go out and about all week. Visiting several resorts, and having picnics on the beach, pub visits and meals of course. They said that Ian had enjoyed himself, and had a video to prove it. When Ian got home he was so happy and sang away all afternoon. The holiday must have worn him out, though, as he slept late over the weekend.

Sunday lunch time Roy and the children came to collect the motor caravan, which he was borrowing to go to France for five weeks' holiday. Paula was to join them later. The caravanette was one of the large ones and I didn't like it, I always found it a pain to drive, but Roy loved it. I had tried a caravan as well, but I was never happy with that either. We liked the idea of our own space. If Ian had a fit while we were travelling or away from home, the caravanette was much better for laying him down or making a drink for him.

July 25 was our 39th wedding anniversary so we took Ian out for a meal in Broadway. Then we began to think about how we were going to celebrate our Ruby wedding. We decided to book a function room at a pub and have the catering done. We held a coffee evening at home on the following Thursday in aid of the new Mencap home. We did quite well - our takings for the day were £213. It was very hectic, but Ian enjoyed having so many people about.

We were finding that Ian was becoming more aware and

capable, wanting to do things like sawing or chopping wood, or knocking nails in. It was nice to see him taking an interest in doing things. Ever the pessimist, I was worrying if it would make him more unsettled when he went to live in the new home, which was now moving forwards. The plans had been drawn and were awaiting final approval. The committee were planning the furniture we would require. We had several offers of financial help, but most of them wanted us to put it to some specific thing. Depending on the amount, we were able to do this as there were several essential items that we needed, from a stair lift at the top end to things like the television or music centre. It has taken over five years to get to this stage. A lot of the delay was down to the county council prevaricating over the new road entrance. The old saying that the mills of the gods run slow but exceedingly small has nothing on the county council. I think they tie a ton weight on all the paperwork to slow it down. Every time it moves on the next person who has to deal with it is either on holiday or off sick. So progress was slow. It put off the day when Ian would leave home, which was good in one way; but in others it was frustrating, dealing with petty officialdom and empire builders.

CHAPTER TWENTY-FIVE

Every time we took Ian to Malvern for the weekend, we worried about him leaving home when the time came. He was always very subdued, which made it difficult for us to leave him. We would probably not have taken him so often if we had not been trying to get him used to being away from home. We did, however, take every advantage of the opportunity to have a break. The weekend Roy and the girls came home from France, Julie also came down with Karma for a few days. We had a few days with them all before we collected Ian, which was nice. It gave Ian a lot of pleasure when saw that the family were home, and Margaret and I felt guilty for not having him home earlier. Daft, isn't it?

We went to our land at Bishampton while they were all here, to plant a load of daffodils. Ian was on holiday from the centre the rest of the time that Julie was here, so I took him round the jobs with me to give Margaret more time with Julie and Karma. The following Saturday Ian was going to Malvern for five days, so we decided to take the caravanette to Devon for a few days. The weather was nice but the caravanette broke down when we tried to leave the site. We had the RAC come to look at it, but they found that the head had warped so they had to tow it to a local garage to get it repaired. We had to get a B & B for two nights while they did the work, then had a bill for £280 for the repairs - not a cheap holiday.

When we collected Ian, although they said he had been fine, we could see how stressed out he was. His psoriasis was worse and his skin was red and angry. It took a few days' careful treatment to calm it down. The following weekend we had a lot of company as Uncle Maurice came with his family. Maurice is much the same age as I am and we were mates when we were young, still are for that matter, so he is more like Ian's uncle. Then one of Julie's friends from Bristol called, with his wife and new baby, and Ian enjoyed himself with all the company.

My Aunt Dora had died and we were going to the funeral on Tuesday 15 September. It's always a sad time when one of the family dies and I am sure Ian missed her; not that he understood, but he still talked about her. As Maurice said, 'We only seem to see some of the family at funerals these days' and I think he was right. It seems such a shame that you seem to drift apart from family and friends as the years pass. I think it's part of the modern way of life, with everyone being in such a rush and moving around the country. Still, I suppose we are the generation who started it all, so perhaps I shouldn't grumble.

The weekend of 21 September Roy and Paula came down with the girls. Unfortunately Ian had a very bad fit in the early hours of Saturday morning and as a consequence was sleepy all day. He only recovered by the evening, when we were ready to go out for a meal. It was Roy and Paula's wedding anniversary on the 19th and we were taking them all out to celebrate it. On the Sunday we took the girls to Mrs Bomford's to have a riding lesson. She hadn't seen Ian for years and couldn't get over how big he was. After lunch they all went back to Manchester. Then later in the week Ian started asking questions like 'Who came to see Ian' or 'Where did Ian went?' It was nice to think that he was remembering what he had been doing. It does not seem like much, but to us it was a big step forward, after years of getting little or no response.

One of the things that Ian loved was having a bath or shower, and at the day centre one of his training programmes was showering and dressing himself. At home we tried to do the same and get him to dress himself after his shower. It was a very slow process and required a lot of patience. When I showered Ian Margaret usually ended up helping him with his dressing, or I dressed him myself as

I soon ran out of patience. I have a great deal of admiration for those who work with handicapped people. I could never do it. It's a completely different matter when you are dealing with one of your own children, but even then Margaret had most of the responsibility.

We had a sort of routine most weekends. If Ian was well enough to go out we would have a look round the shops, then have lunch out, the highlight of the day for Ian. The Saturday after Roy and family went home, we went out as usual. As luck would have it we were back home fairly early, for just as we arrived home a friend from California turned up on his motorbike. Had we been late, as we often were, we would have missed him.

I had met John Huegel at the Vincent international rally and whenever he was in England he would call and stop for a couple of nights. On this occasion, he had ridden to Greece with some of the Vincent Club and he called to see us before flying home. We always have an open house, in fact we have often asked complete strangers in for a coffee if we have seen them looking around the village at the maypole and thatched cottages. We feel so lucky to live in such a pleasant place, especially when we talk to strangers and find that they live in the city. I suppose that some people might worry about their security, inviting strangers in, but we have always had two or three strong dogs in the house who are very protective of the family. Anyway, Ian always enjoyed company, whether he knew the people or not.

At the beginning of October we asked if we could see the video that the staff had taken of Ian's summer holiday. We arranged to see it at one of their open days and were looking forward to it. Ian started the month very chatty and alert most of the time, although when we took him to the cinema to see Goldie Hawn in The House Sitter, he slept through most of the film. The manager of our local cinema still insisted on not letting us pay for Ian, which we always appreciated.

The new home (no name yet) was grinding slowly forward and we were expecting a starting date for the construction in the near future. Margaret and I were getting butterflies in our tummies at the thought of it. Margaret had started to write down all of Ian's likes and dislikes, as she felt that they may not understand his behaviour, or what he said and meant. We wanted to have him home at the weekends, but this also worried us in case it affected the way he settled down.

Ian had a bad cold one week and it got worse as the week wore on, so he had a week at home being pampered. Luckily he didn't have too many fits, as he did sometimes when he was unwell. By the weekend he was much better and brighter, though he required much more reassurance about things.

On the 18th of the month Julie and Steve came down with baby Karma to take the caravanette to Scotland. They wanted to leave it by their new house up in the mountains while they were working on it, so they would have somewhere to look after Karma. Roy and his family also came down for the weekend as we were having the girls for part of the half term so Roy could get on with some studying while Paula was at work. (He had decided to carry on with his studies after getting his maths degree.) All the family were here together for a change, and Margaret could spend plenty time with them. Grandmothers have more time than they did when their own children were young.

It was very much of a rush in the mornings getting Ian ready to go to the day centre, as well as looking after the girls. However, once the mini bus and escort collected Ian, things calmed down a little. I was soon off to work so Margaret had to amuse the girls on her own. Then of course by 4pm it was all go again when Ian arrived home, wanting his tea as usual.

On Wednesday afternoon, 21 October 1991, Roy collected the girls and headed home, as he had an exam the next day. Ian was sad that Roy was leaving, but soon accepted it. We got him ready for bed around 11pm and he soon settled. Little did we know that our lives were to change so dramatically in just a few hours.

CHAPTER TWENTY-SIX

Just before 5am on the 22 October, we heard Ian having a fit. There was the usual panic as we stumbled out of bed and almost fell down the stairs in a rush to get to his room. He was still fitting as we got to him, so we turned him onto his side as we always did. When he came out of the fit, we tried to settle him down but he became very disorientated and wanted to get up. Sometimes during a very bad fit he would wet the bed, in which case we would have to get him up to change the sheets. At other times he would just want to turn over and he would be asleep before we could get out of the room. Then at other times he would be very disorientated and want to go to the kitchen. When he settled, we would make him a cup of tea and after a while he would go back to bed and sleep for a long time. But on this occasion, as I helped him along the bed and we got to the end, Ian just slipped to the floor. I told Margaret to ring the ambulance as he was going into a fit again. She rang 999 and when she came back, I was sat on the floor with Ian in my arms. I said, 'He's gone, love.' Margaret screamed, 'No! no!' We tried to revive him, then the ambulance arrived. I think I knew it was too late, because Ian looked so peaceful; I had never seen his face so serene.

The next two hours were a nightmare come true. The ambulance men were wonderful. They tried to revive him, but to no avail. They came out and said that Ian had died. It was then that I had these horrible feelings of guilt, thinking that we could have done more to save him. I asked if they were going to take Ian to the hospital, but they said they were not allowed to and would have to wait until the doctor and the police arrived.

Our local GP, Dr Smith, arrived and examined Ian before certifying him dead. He was absolutely marvellous; he stood by the Aga hugging both Margaret and me (it's nearly seven years ago and I am crying trying to write this now). We will never forget the support that Dr Smith gave at such a terrible time. The vicar also called by about 7.30am: I never did find out how he knew that Ian had died. A policeman was the next to arrive, then the ambulance men were able to leave. I only wish I could say something nice about the police constable who came, but he showed no sympathy at all. The only thing that interested him was using our phone to ring the police station every ten minutes, complaining that he was off duty at 6am and this was a job for the sergeant. When he was not on the phone he was telling us it was not his job. It wasn't until the undertakers arrived to take Ian to the coroner that he even asked me to identify Ian.

After they had taken Ian away, Margaret and I both had to make a statement to the policeman. Finally, when we were alone, I realised that I would have to start phoning everyone to let them know. We were in shock, running on auto pilot, not really knowing what we were doing. After considering if we should tell Roy before his exam, I thought it was better that he knew, so I rang him at about 8.30. He wanted to come straight down but we told him that there was little he could do and we wanted him to take his exam. Then I rang Julie, but she was so far away that we told her not to come for a couple of days. When I rang Pat she got a lift and came over, then Annie came from over the road and stayed till tea time. It took a long time to phone all out friends and relatives, as I had to brace myself between each call.

During the morning I heard the church bells ringing. They always ring the bells in the village very slowly when someone dies, and it is nice as it shows that others care. Some of our neighbours called by during the day and in the evening to offer their condolences, which helped us a lot.

My brother David and his wife Carol came over after lunch -

not that we could eat any - and brought Margot with them. They stayed with us for a couple of hours, then at tea time Pat and Anne went home and Anthony and Jane from next door came round to see how we were. They asked if we wanted to be alone or needed company. We said that we would like them to stay, and they did, until after 3am. They brought a bottle of scotch with them and we drank it before they went home. We are not used to strong drink, so I think it must have been the scotch that finally put us to sleep for a couple of hours.

The next day the coroner rang to say he would not be asking for an inquest and he would issue the death certificate, so we could arrange the funeral. I asked if Ian's heart had failed, but he said that his heart was as sound as a bell. I said I thought that all the fits he had would have weakened it, but he said that, as the heart is a muscle, the fits would have strengthened it. He said that he would be putting the cause of death down as a/ Status Epilepticus, b/ Cerebral Atrophy after post-mortem without inquest. We know this is incorrect as we were with him when he died, so we know he was not in status; he had come out of the fit for several minutes before he died. It is only later, when you have time to reflect, that you look at things like that more carefully.

The care and concern that our friends like Pat showed at our worst time are things we will never, ever forget. Roy arrived on the Friday; Paula and the girls would come down later for the funeral. Then the funeral director rang to say that Ian was in their chapel if anyone wanted to see him. Margaret wanted to go so we went and he still looked peaceful, just as if he was asleep. We needed to go as the tears we shed there were something of a relief. A lot of people said, 'You are being brave' but in actual fact everything was passing us by in a blur. I suppose we were in shock for the first two or three weeks. It's nature's way of helping you over what is probably the worst thing that can happen to you.

Julie arrived with Karma on the Monday, Steve was following later. She wanted to see Ian so we went with her. We wished we hadn't gone because Ian didn't look as good as when we first saw him. With all our family and friends around us we were getting by.

Our next hurdle would be the funeral, which was to be on Thursday 30 October. We had to go into the registry office in Evesham to register Ian's death, then make all the funeral arrangements, like sorting out the service and what hymns we wanted. It was a busy time, but I think this helps as you don't have too much time to brood.

On the day of the funeral, they brought Ian home in the hearse and we all walked behind it to the church. It was like walking through a fog; nothing about that day was very clear. The thing that sticks in my mind most was looking round the church and being amazed at the amount of people there. It was full to overflowing with family, friends and neighbours, including several of the staff and Ian's friends from the day centre. There were so many people that a lot of them had to stand. After they had buried Ian, Margaret and I stood by the churchyard gate to thank everyone for coming, and invite them to the cottage. Pat and Annie had spent the morning preparing all the food, so there was plenty to eat and drink.

Ian is buried in the lovely village churchyard, only 300-400 yards from our cottage. It's a very pretty place with a riot of flowers all the year round. You can sit there at peace with the world. It was a great help having Roy, Julie and our grandchildren around us, but they had their own lives to lead. So a couple of days after the funeral we were on our own and starting to realise what had happened to us.

We did and still do feel lost without Ian. He was so totally dependant on us for so long that we formed an indescribable bond. It's easy for people to think, 'Well, now he's at peace at last and you're free to lead your own lives.' It's not like that in reality. Our grief was even too deep to cry at the time; you just learn how to behave in public. We still go to the day centre from time and a few months after losing Ian the staff gave us a copy of the videos they had made of Ian. Every time we went they would ask if we had watched them, but we had to say no. That, is until last Christmas. We see the children and grandchildren just before and just after Christmas, but we like to spend Christmas Day on our with our memories. So last Christmas we plucked up courage and watched the videos of our Ian. Even through our tears we enjoyed watching him, and we actually felt happy.

In the first few weeks after losing Ian we collected all the photos we could find of him and sorted out the ones we liked the best. We had some enlargements done and placed them around the house, so he is always with us. We didn't do too many but enough to see him as we move about the house. We also had to sort out his clothes. Ian had a lot of good quality clothes, so we parcelled most of them up and took them to the Salvation Army. We asked for them to go to the homeless in Britain, not abroad. Ian's bedroom is still the same as when he used it, but it has not become a shrine. We do use it when the family come to stay and over the years Roy and most of the grandchildren have slept there. Probably the room we now use most is the little sun room that we did up for Ian. I retired nearly five years ago and we now sit there every day, watching the birds and admiring the garden.

Hippy, our Alsatian who followed Ian everywhere, was only eight years old when she was taken ill a few days after Ian's death. She went downhill fast. Less than three weeks after we lost Ian, she was so weak that I had to carry her into the vet's. He tried his best to save her but the last time we took her he said: 'If you don't let me put her to sleep now, you'll regret it by tomorrow, as she is suffering and I can't do any more for her.' Margaret and I held her in our arms, crying our eyes out, while the vet put her to sleep. We have always felt that she lost the will to live when Ian had gone. We had her cremated so we could lay her to rest with all our other dogs at the top of our garden.

By now we were wondering what else could happen, and sure enough, a few weeks later we lost our little Jack Russell, Toby. However, he was over 17 years old, so it wasn't totally unexpected. Then poor Pippin, our Staffordshire, caused us concern as she was pining for her two mates. With a lot of affection she started to improve and thankfully went on for some time.

We cannot remember much of the first 12 months after Ian died. It was like walking down a black tunnel with no light at the end. We carried on from day to day on autopilot, hardly noticing what was going on. But gradually you start to come back to life, although your life has changed forever. I am much more demonstrative now than I have ever been. If I watch something on TV or read in the paper about some tragedy, I get quite emotional.

The contract for the new home had now started and I decided that I would like to stay involved in the project, in Ian's memory. We were finally ready to open in April of 1994, and at the official opening, both Margaret and me shed a few tears. It was nice that it had finally opened. I talked our Pat into applying for one of the care assistants' jobs and she turned out to be a natural. The only thing that worries me is that if anything happens to any of them she will break her heart.

Just over two years after Ian died, I decided to retire as I was 67. The following spring the Vincent Club was having an international rally in New Zealand for three weeks, so we decided to go. After booking the trip I kept thinking of other places I would like us to see. Margaret was frightened to let me out of her sight, in case I came back having extended our trip yet again!

We ended up going to Los Angeles, Honolulu, Fiji, then New Zealand for three weeks. From there we went to Australia for four weeks. We came home via Thailand, India and Nepal. The only place we have been since is the Orkneys, and although we are glad that we have seen all these places, it has made us realise how lucky we are to live where we do and we have no ambitions for further travel.

On our land at Bishampton where we planted all those trees, we put a plaque up dedicating the land as a nature reserve to Ian's memory. We also wanted to plant a tree or put a seat in the churchyard in Ian's memory. The church was not keen on us doing that, but asked if we would replace the broken cross over the porch. It was a stone cross, four feet tall with the one arm broken off, so there was plenty left to copy. As it was in Cotswold stone, I erected some scaffolding, removed the old cross and took it to the quarry at the top of Broadway Hill, where they carved a new one to match the original. A few weeks later I collected it and fitted it over the church porch. Now it has had time to weather it looks as if it has been there for many years.

Despite all our problems over the years, we would never have been without our Ian. We still had a full life with a lot of pleasure and fun. So for anyone who is in the same position as we were all that time ago, we can only say: stick with it, because when things are at their blackest they can only get better. There is greater tolerance out there now and more help than there was 40 years ago, as long as things don't slip back. This could happen, as the latest tendency to cut Social Services is very worrying, especially the cutting back of day care in Worcestershire. With the government awash with money, you would think things would get better but there are times when I despair.

But enough moaning for now. Life goes on. We always tell Ian what is going on when we attend to his grave and change his flowers. If anyone thinks we are odd when they hear us talking to him, we don't give a damn; it gives us some comfort. As I come to the end of our little family saga, all that remains is to thank the reader for seeing it through to the end. Thank you.

Contact Addresses

SUDEP
Epilepsy Bereaved
P.O. Box 112
Wantage
OX12 8XT
Telephone: 01235 772850

British Epilepsy Association
New Anstey House Gateway Drive
Yeadon
Leeds LS19 7XY
Telephone: 0113 218 8800
Email: epilepsy@bea.org.uk
Website: www.epilepsy.org.uk

The National Autistic Society
393 City Road
London EC1V 1NG
Telephone: 020 7833 2299
Email: nas@nas.org.uk
Website: www.oneworld.org/autism-uk

MENCAP
123 Golden Lane
London
EC1Y 0RT
Telephone: 020 7454 0454
Website: http://www.mencap.org.uk/

Bereavement Contact Line: 01235 772852
General Inquiries and Fax: 01235 772850
E-mail: epilepsybereaved@dial.pipex.com
http://dspace.dial.pipex.com/epilepsybereaved/

Lionel Wilkes
Email: Lionel3@tesco.net
Website: http:/homepages.tesco.net/~lionel3/index.html